NATIONAL ACADEMIES *Sciences Engineering Medicine*

NATIONAL
ACADEMIES
PRESS
Washington, DC

Use of Meta-Analyses in Nutrition Research and Policy

Melissa Maitin-Shepard and Marian Flaxman, *Rapporteurs*

Food and Nutrition Board

Health and Medicine Division

Proceedings of a Workshop Series

NATIONAL ACADEMIES PRESS 500 Fifth Street, NW Washington, DC 20001

This activity was supported by a contract between the National Academy of Sciences and the U.S. Food and Drug Administration. Any opinions, findings, conclusions, or recommendations expressed in this publication do not necessarily reflect the views of any organization or agency that provided support for the project.

International Standard Book Number-13: 978-0-309-71579-9
International Standard Book Number-10: 0-309-71579-2
Digital Object Identifier: https://doi.org/10.17226/27481

This publication is available from the National Academies Press, 500 Fifth Street, NW, Keck 360, Washington, DC 20001; (800) 624-6242 or (202) 334-3313; http://www.nap.edu.

Copyright 2024 by the National Academy of Sciences. National Academies of Sciences, Engineering, and Medicine and National Academies Press and the graphical logos for each are all trademarks of the National Academy of Sciences. All rights reserved.

Printed in the United States of America.

Suggested citation: National Academies of Sciences, Engineering, and Medicine. 2024. *Use of meta-analyses in nutrition research and policy: Proceedings of a workshop series.* Washington, DC: The National Academies Press. https://doi.org/10.17226/27481.

The **National Academy of Sciences** was established in 1863 by an Act of Congress, signed by President Lincoln, as a private, nongovernmental institution to advise the nation on issues related to science and technology. Members are elected by their peers for outstanding contributions to research. Dr. Marcia McNutt is president.

The **National Academy of Engineering** was established in 1964 under the charter of the National Academy of Sciences to bring the practices of engineering to advising the nation. Members are elected by their peers for extraordinary contributions to engineering. Dr. John L. Anderson is president.

The **National Academy of Medicine** (formerly the Institute of Medicine) was established in 1970 under the charter of the National Academy of Sciences to advise the nation on medical and health issues. Members are elected by their peers for distinguished contributions to medicine and health. Dr. Victor J. Dzau is president.

The three Academies work together as the **National Academies of Sciences, Engineering, and Medicine** to provide independent, objective analysis and advice to the nation and conduct other activities to solve complex problems and inform public policy decisions. The National Academies also encourage education and research, recognize outstanding contributions to knowledge, and increase public understanding in matters of science, engineering, and medicine.

Learn more about the National Academies of Sciences, Engineering, and Medicine at **www.nationalacademies.org**.

Consensus Study Reports published by the National Academies of Sciences, Engineering, and Medicine document the evidence-based consensus on the study's statement of task by an authoring committee of experts. Reports typically include findings, conclusions, and recommendations based on information gathered by the committee and the committee's deliberations. Each report has been subjected to a rigorous and independent peer-review process and it represents the position of the National Academies on the statement of task.

Proceedings published by the National Academies of Sciences, Engineering, and Medicine chronicle the presentations and discussions at a workshop, symposium, or other event convened by the National Academies. The statements and opinions contained in proceedings are those of the participants and are not endorsed by other participants, the planning committee, or the National Academies.

Rapid Expert Consultations published by the National Academies of Sciences, Engineering, and Medicine are authored by subject-matter experts on narrowly focused topics that can be supported by a body of evidence. The discussions contained in rapid expert consultations are considered those of the authors and do not contain policy recommendations. Rapid expert consultations are reviewed by the institution before release.

For information about other products and activities of the National Academies, please visit www.nationalacademies.org/about/whatwedo.

PLANNING COMMITTEE FOR THE WORKSHOP SERIES ON THE USE OF META-ANALYSES IN NUTRITION RESEARCH AND POLICY

KATHERINE L. TUCKER (*Chair*), University Distinguished Professor of Nutritional Epidemiology in the Department of Biomedical and Nutrition Sciences and Director of the Center for Population Health, University of Massachusetts Lowell

MEI CHUNG, Professor, Gerold J. and Dorothy R. Friedman School of Nutrition Science and Policy, Tufts University

RUSSELL JUDE DE SOUZA, Professor, Department of Health Research Methods, Evidence, and Impact, McMaster University

AMANDA J. MacFARLANE, Founding Director of the Agriculture, Food, and Nutrition Evidence Center and Professor of Nutrition, Texas A&M University

CHIZURU NISHIDA, Head of the Cross-Cutting Unit of Safe, Healthy and Sustainable Diets, Department of Nutrition and Food Safety, World Health Organization (retired); Chair, Cochrane Nutrition Advisory Board (*until 2023*)

JANET A. TOOZE, Professor, Department of Biostatistics and Data Science, Division of Public Health Sciences, Wake Forest University School of Medicine

Staff

TAKYERA ROBINSON, Associate Program Officer (*until November 2023*)

ALICE VOROSMARTI, Associate Program Officer (*from November 2023*)

SAMUEL CRAWFORD, Senior Program Assistant

ANN L. YAKTINE, Director, Food and Nutrition Board

Rapporteurs

MELISSA MAITIN-SHEPARD, MMS Health Strategies, LLC

MARIAN FLAXMAN, Informed Solutions, LLC

Reviewers

This Proceedings of a Workshop Series was reviewed in draft form by individuals chosen for their diverse perspectives and technical expertise. The purpose of this independent review is to provide candid and critical comments that will assist the National Academies of Sciences, Engineering, and Medicine in making each published proceedings as sound as possible and to ensure that it meets the institutional standards for quality, objectivity, evidence, and responsiveness to the charge. The review comments and draft manuscript remain confidential to protect the integrity of the process.

We thank the following individuals for their review of this proceedings:

MARTHA FIELD, Cornell University
PAULE JOSEPH, National Institutes of Health, National Institute on
    Alcohol Abuse and Alcoholism
KATHERINE TUCKER, University of Massachusetts Lowell

Although the reviewers listed above provided many constructive comments and suggestions, they were not asked to endorse the content of the proceedings nor did they see the final draft before its release. The review of this proceedings was overseen by **CELINE HESKEY,** Loma Linda University. She was responsible for making certain that an independent examination of this proceedings was carried out in accordance with standards of the National Academies and that all review comments were carefully considered. Responsibility for the final content rests entirely with the rapporteurs and the National Academies.

Contents

ACRONYMS AND ABBREVIATIONS xiii

1 INTRODUCTION 1
Overview of the Workshop Series, 4
Opening Remarks from Workshop Sponsor, 5

2 PLANNING OF SYSTEMATIC REVIEWS AND
META-ANALYSES 7
Planning for Systematic Reviews and Meta-Analyses, 8
Methods for Reducing the Risk of Bias in Systematic Reviews
and Meta-Analyses, 12
Panel Discussion, 19

3 EXPLORING BEST PRACTICES OF CONDUCTING
META-ANALYSIS 25
Best Practices of Meta-Analysis in Nutrition Research, 26
Interpreting the Results of Meta-Analyses and Addressing
Heterogeneity, 34
Panel Discussion, 43

4   INTERPRETATION AND APPLICATION OF SYSTEMATIC
    REVIEWS AND META-ANALYSIS TO EVALUATE THE
    TOTALITY OF EVIDENCE   49
    From Science to Policy: Evaluating Nutrition Evidence
        for Informed Decision Making, 50
    Nutrition and Policy: Evaluating the Evidence, 59
    Panel Discussion, 64

5   CLOSING REMARKS   69
    Takeaways from the Workshop Series,

REFERENCES   71

APPENDIXES
A   Workshop Agendas   73
B   Speaker and Moderator Biographies   77

Boxes, Figures, and Table

BOXES

1-1   Statement of Task, 2

4-1   PICO for Health Canada's Systematic Review on Whole Grain Intake and Coronary Heart Disease, 57

FIGURES

3-1   An example of a data extraction template, 28
3-2   An example of a funnel plot used to identify publication bias, 32
3-3   An example of a GOSH analysis of an influential study, 35
3-4   Forest plot for a systematic review of low-sodium salt substitutes and diastolic blood pressure, 37
3-5   Equations used in the fixed effects and random effects models, 38
3-6   An example of rating risk of bias through color coding in a forest plot, 41

4-1   A systematic approach to health claims substantiation, 52
4-2   Potential types of bias in nutrition studies, 54
4-3   Quality appraisal tool for intervention studies and quality appraisal tool for prospective observational studies used by Health Canada, 55

4-4   USDA NESR's process for structuring a systematic review, 62
4-5   A hierarchy of evidence for health claims substantiation used
       by Health Canada, 66

TABLE

2-1   Limitations in Observational Studies, 15

Acronyms and Abbreviations

AI   artificial intelligence

CHD   coronary heart disease
CI   confidence interval

DGA   *Dietary Guidelines for Americans*
DGAC   Dietary Guidelines Advisory Committee

FDA   U.S. Food and Drug Administration
FSN   fail-safe N

GOSH   Graphical Display of Study Heterogeneity
GRADE   Grading of Recommendations, Assessment, Development
            and Evaluation

LSSS   low-sodium salt substitutes

MA   meta-analysis

NESR   Nutrition Evidence Systematic Review
NOS   Newcastle-Ottawa Scale
NUGAG   Nutrition Guidance Expert Advisory Group

PICO   Population, Intervention, Comparator, Outcome
PRISMA   Preferred Reporting Items for Systematic Reviews and
             Meta-Analyses

RCT   randomized controlled trial
ROBINS-E   Risk of Bias in Non-randomized Studies–of Exposures
ROBINS-I   Risk of Bias in Non-randomized Studies–of Interventions
ROBIS   Risk of Bias in Systematic Reviews

SF   saturated fat
SR   systematic review

USDA   U.S. Department of Agriculture

WHO   World Health Organization

1

Introduction[1]

In September and October 2023, the National Academies of Sciences, Engineering, and Medicine's (the National Academies') Food and Nutrition Board held a three-part virtual workshop series to discuss best practices for conducting meta-analyses (MAs) in nutrition research and utilizing MAs to inform policy. The three-part series, titled Use of Meta-Analyses in Nutrition Research and Policy: A Workshop Series, explored the evidence on methods for conducting, interpreting, and integrating the results of MAs for use in nutrition research, developing nutrition policy, and informing nutrition regulatory decision making.

The workshop series was sponsored by the U.S. Food and Drug Administration (FDA) and featured invited presentations and discussions with researchers, government officials, and other global leaders in nutrition research and policy. The workshop Statement of Task can be found in Box 1-1. The agendas for each workshop are presented in Appendix A, and Appendix B contains the biographical sketches of the speakers and moderators.

The workshop series included three 2-hour workshops that took place over a 3-week period and was planned by a committee, which was led by Katherine L. Tucker of the University of Massachusetts Lowell and

---

[1] The planning committee's role was limited to planning the workshop, and the Proceedings of a Workshop was prepared by the workshop rapporteurs as a factual summary of what occurred at the workshop. Statements, recommendations, and opinions expressed are those of individual presenters and participants, and are not necessarily endorsed or verified by the National Academies of Sciences, Engineering, and Medicine, and they should not be construed as reflecting any group consensus.

BOX 1-1
Statement of Task

A planning committee of the National Academies of Sciences, Engineering, and Medicine will organize a series of virtual public workshops that explore the evidence on methods for conducting, interpreting, and integrating the results of meta-analyses for use in nutrition research, developing nutrition policy, and informing nutrition regulatory decision making. The workshops will feature invited presentations and discussions that will focus on improving guidance to researchers and policy makers. Specific topic areas to be considered include:

- Criteria used to determine clinical or methodological differences among individual nutrition studies;
- Extraction errors and errors in calculating mean differences and confidence intervals from the primary studies that are included in a meta-analysis;
- Benchmark practices for planning appropriate subgroup and sensitivity analyses and addressing publication bias;
- Use of meta-analyses to evaluate the strength of the totality of evidence;
- Interpretation and integration of meta-analyses and direction of effect of individual studies into the overall body of evidence;
- Evaluation of the strength of the evidence when different outcomes are reported in different studies;
- Consideration of statistical heterogeneity and risk of bias when evaluating diet and disease relationships; and
- Communication of meta-analyses relevant to nutrition policy decision makers.

The planning committee will select and invite speakers and discussants as well as moderate the discussions. A workshop proceedings will be prepared by a designated rapporteur in accordance with institutional guidelines.

---

comprised of leading experts in nutrition research and policy. Prior to the workshop series, FDA staff provided the planning committee with a list of questions to be addressed throughout the workshops. The questions for the first workshop are:

- What are best practices in identifying and avoiding extraction errors and errors in calculating mean differences and confidence intervals from the primary studies that are included in an MA, given that these errors are common in published literature?
- How should an MA be evaluated for methodological quality when extraction and/or data errors are present? At what point do data

errors (in kind and number) reach a level that invalidates the conclusions of the MA?

- How to consider risk of bias when evaluating diet and disease relationships?
- What are the best practices for addressing publication bias?
- What criteria should be used to determine whether individual nutrition studies have too many clinical or methodological differences (e.g., treatment, dose, population, mean body mass index, duration, comparators/diets, results) to be combined into the same MA?
- What are best practices for planning appropriate subgroups and sensitivity analysis a priori?
- How can MA be used to evaluate the strength of the evidence when different outcomes are reported in different studies? And how can MA be used to evaluate the strength of the totality of evidence?

The questions for the second workshop are:

- Extraction errors from the primary studies that are included in MAs are common. What are best practices for avoiding/identifying these types of errors?
- What are the best practices for addressing publication bias?

The questions for the third workshop are:

- How to consider statistical heterogeneity when evaluating diet and disease relationships? Are higher levels of unexplained statistical heterogeneity acceptable for the field of nutrition? What are the best practices for addressing publication bias?
- How to consider risk of bias when evaluating diet and disease relationships?
- How can MA be used to evaluate the strength of the totality of evidence when there is evidence from different types of nutrition study designs?
- How can MA be used to evaluate the strength of evidence when different outcomes are reported in different studies?

As previously stated, the goals of the workshop series were to explore issues and best practices around MA. However, because MAs and systematic reviews (SRs) are closely related processes, they share many of the same important considerations. In light of this, many presentations included broader discussions around issues related to both MAs and SRs.

OVERVIEW OF THE WORKSHOP SERIES

The first workshop in the series, held on September 19, 2023, focused on the planning and execution of MAs for nutrition research. Workshop objectives included clarifying criteria for the selection of studies to be included in an MA, with a focus on the Population, Intervention, Comparator, and Outcome (PICO) framework, and planning for subgroup analyses. The agenda for the first workshop included opening remarks from planning committee chair Katherine L. Tucker, background information on the topic and the goals for the workshop, presentations from invited speakers Crystal Rivers and Sarah Gebauer from FDA, Celeste Naude of Stellenbosch University, and Lee Hooper of the University of East Anglia, and a panel discussion featuring Hooper, Naude, and additional discussants. Naude guided participants through the planning of SRs and MAs and addressed topics such as how SRs and MAs can be used to evaluate the strength of the evidence when different outcomes are reported in different studies. In the second presentation, Hooper focused on the pillars of planning that can help reduce the risk of bias in an SR or MA. Through this lens, Hooper addressed topics of how to consider risk of bias when evaluating diet and disease relationships and the best practices for addressing publication bias. The panel discussion featured additional discussants, including Sydne Newberry of the RAND Corporation and Christopher Schmid of the Brown University School of Public Health. The discussion was moderated by planning committee member Amanda J. MacFarlane of Texas A&M University. The closing remarks for this first workshop were delivered by planning committee member Mei Chung of Tufts University.

The second workshop featured presentations on best practices in conducting SRs and MAs, especially in the context of nutrition research and policy development. The objectives for the session were to explain the best practices for screening data for potential errors, how to use a system of evaluation for understanding risk of bias in study design, and how to systematically evaluate study results, including understanding the precision of estimates and the potential for publication bias. Finally, the workshop explored how to effectively interpret the results of an MA using a variety of statistical methods, what to do if assumptions are violated, and how to address the issue of high statistical heterogeneity, which is common in nutrition studies. The agenda for the 2-hour workshop included presentations from Emma Boyland of the University of Liverpool, Andrew Jones of Liverpool John Moores University, and George A. Wells of the University of Ottawa. Following the presentations, a panel discussion featured the presenters and additional discussants. The discussion included questions and contributions from Elie A. Akl from the American University of Beirut, Joseph Beyene of McMaster University, and M. Hassan Murad of the Mayo

Clinic. The discussion was moderated by planning committee member Janet A. Tooze of the Wake Forest University School of Medicine, and closing remarks were given by planning committee member Russell Jude de Souza of McMaster University.

The third and final workshop in the series featured presentations on best practices in interpretation and application of SRs and MAs, especially in the context of nutrition research. The objectives of the session were to recognize the impact of risk of bias and publication bias on the interpretation of study results, to describe the impact of data errors on the conclusions of SRs and MAs, to describe the process of evaluating the strength of the totality of evidence, to describe the different applications of SRs and MAs to research and policy, and to consider the evidence evaluation for each. The 2-hour workshop included presentations from Karima Benkhedda of Health Canada and Barbara O. Schneeman of the University of California, Davis. Following the presentations, a panel discussion, moderated by planning committee member Chizuru Nishida of the World Health Organization, retired, featured remarks from the presenters as well as Vasanti Malik from the University of Toronto and Elie A. Akl from the American University of Beirut. Closing remarks were given by Katherine L. Tucker. She also presented the final remarks for the entire workshop series.

Although each workshop had a distinct focus, several topics were reiterated throughout the series. For example, Hooper discussed ways to examine and reduce risk of bias, and Boyland explored methods of anticipating and avoiding bias in study design. Jones and Wells discussed the many ways in which statistical analyses can fail to address the unique needs of nutrition research, and Schneemann emphasized the benefits of consistent use of statistical tools to improve statistical analysis in the complex field of nutrition research. Discussion also focused on whether the field of nutrition research requires unique tools for evidence synthesis and decision making. In the closing remarks of the workshop series, Tucker noted that the complexities of nutrition research may require distinctive considerations and suggested that the best practices described throughout the series could inform future nutrition research and policy development. She stated that the field of nutrition research is not only uniquely complex but also uniquely situated to have a real-life impact on large populations through evidence-based policy development.

OPENING REMARKS FROM WORKSHOP SPONSOR

At the beginning of the first workshop, two speakers from FDA explained why their agency sponsored the workshop series. One example they gave is that MAs are increasingly reported in the scientific literature in the nutrition field, and stakeholders are increasingly requesting that federal agencies consider MAs in support of nutrition policy and regulatory decisions. Crystal Rivers and Sarah Gebauer each spoke about FDA's investment in the workshop series and the unique research and policy development challenges faced by the field of nutrition.

Rivers spoke about the use of MAs in the development of nutrition regulatory decisions, nutrition policy, and dietary recommendations and how MAs can be used to identify existing gaps in nutrition research. She noted that the use of MAs with SRs is becoming more common and that there has been a lack of discussion around how to best use and conduct MAs in the field of nutrition. Rivers explained that it was the hope of FDA that this workshop series would help inform a set of best practices for the use of MAs in nutrition policy development moving forward.

Gebauer emphasized the unique needs of FDA when it comes to their nutrition regulatory framework and how evidence is used to substantiate health claims by showing a direct relationship between a food product and a health outcome or disease risk. She gave an example of the nutrients calcium and vitamin D and their relationship to osteoporosis. Gebauer noted that when evidence for a health claim is weak, the strength of the evidence must be reflected in the language of the claim. She also pointed out some of FDA's distinctive considerations when conducting their own reviews of the evidence related to nutrition labeling and health claims. For example, FDA typically conducts health claim reviews in response to stakeholder petitions, which identify the topic of the review based on stakeholder interests; and FDA relies on publicly available data for their health claim reviews. Gebauer highlighted the need for consistent application of tools and a set of best practices for conducting MAs and for evaluating and interpreting MAs in nutrition research and policy. She noted that FDA hoped to use the discussions from the workshop series to inform the development of clear recommendations for evaluating the quality of existing MAs, conducting MAs, and interpretating and integrating outcomes of MAs to evaluate the strength of a body of evidence for the development of nutrition policy.

2

Planning of Systematic Reviews and Meta-Analyses

This chapter describes the presentations and discussions that took place during the first workshop, titled Use of Meta-Analyses in Nutrition Research and Policy: Planning of Meta-Analysis, which took place on September 19, 2023. The objectives of the workshop were to

- Apply criteria to select studies for inclusion in systematic reviews (SRs) and meta-analyses (MAs), with a focus on PICO (Population, Intervention [including treatment, dose, duration], Comparators [with consideration of diet], and Outcomes [with consideration for adjustment for confounders/covariates]);
- Account for subgroup and sensitivity analyses when planning an SR and MA; and
- Use an appropriate data management system for extracting data.

Following the opening remarks, planning committee member Amanda J. MacFarlane of Texas A&M University welcomed attendees and introduced the day's two main presenters, Celeste Naude of Stellenbosch University and Lee Hooper of the University of East Anglia. Naude and Hooper's presentations addressed the foundational aspects of planning and delivering a high-quality nutrition SR and MA. Their presentation was divided into two parts, Naude delivering the first section on planning for a successful SR and MA and Hooper speaking about methods for SRs and MAs in the second half. A panel discussion moderated by MacFarlane followed the presentations. The panel included Naude, Hooper, and two additional discussants,

Sydne Newberry of the RAND Corporation and Christopher Schmid from the Brown University School of Public Health.

PLANNING FOR SYSTEMATIC REVIEWS AND META-ANALYSES

Naude and Hooper's presentation was titled "Systematic Reviews & Meta-Analysis for Developing Nutrition Guidance: The Core Pillars of Planning and Methods to Deliver High Quality, Useful Synthesized Evidence." The presentation addressed the following questions, which were posed in advance by the workshop sponsor:

- What are best practices in identifying and avoiding extraction errors and errors in calculating mean differences and confidence intervals from the primary studies that are included in a meta-analysis, given that these errors are common in published literature?
- How should an MA be evaluated for methodological quality when extraction or data errors are present? At what point do data errors (in kind and number) reach a level that invalidates the conclusions of the MA?
- How to consider risk of bias when evaluating diet and disease relationships?
- What are the best practices for addressing publication bias?
- What criteria should be used to determine whether individual nutrition studies have too many clinical or methodological differences (e.g., treatment, dose, population, mean body mass index, duration, comparators/diets, results) to be combined into the same MA?
- What are best practices for planning appropriate subgroups and sensitivity analysis a priori?
- How can MA be used to evaluate the strength of the evidence when different outcomes are reported in different studies? And how can MA be used to evaluate the strength of the totality of evidence?

Naude began by providing a brief overview of the presentation topics. She noted the importance of the planning phase of an SR or MA and how the planning process can set up a research team for success. Naude framed her involvement in the field of nutrition research, noting that she is the codirector of Cochrane Nutrition and is involved in other Cochrane groups. She is also a founding member of the South Africa Grading of Recommendations, Assessment, Development and Evaluation (GRADE) Network. GRADE is a research tool used to develop and present summaries of evidence and provide a systematic and transparent approach for assessing the certainty (or quality) of the evidence and making recommendations. Naude stated that she receives no industry funding. As she introduced the topics and content of her presentation, Naude contextualized that much of the content had been guided by the latest online version of the *Cochrane Handbook for Systematic Reviews of Interventions, version 6.4* (updated August 2023).[1]

Naude explained the basic concepts of SRs and MAs. She stated that while many people confuse the two, there are important differences between them and they can be effectively used in conjunction with each other. An SR is a well-defined and described research method, and an MA is a method of statistical analysis, which may be part of the SR process. SRs pull together the results of many primary studies that meet pre-specified criteria to answer clear and well-framed research questions and are used to minimize bias when reviewing and assessing evidence. The analysis and interpretations used in an SR consider the internal validity of the studies involved and additional factors that may impact the certainty of the evidence. Naude stated that SRs should be performed in rigorous, methodological ways to reduce reviewer selection bias, and should have pre-determined rules for identifying and including studies.

As Naude described, an MA is a statistical method that may be part of the SR process. She emphasized that all MAs should be informed by a rigorous SR. Naude explained that MAs combine the numerical results of studies[2] (e.g., mean differences, odds ratios, risk ratios, or confidence intervals) and require transparency and careful planning. The results of an MA, as well as an SR, can be misleading if the underlying methods are not sound. Naude explained that setting up an SR or MA with clear questions and methods a priori is essential for minimizing bias and improving the reliability of the results. Naude acknowledged that conducting SRs and MAs can be time consuming and complex but reiterated that completing them correctly is essential because, when done right, they can be useful tools in the development of evidence-based policies and guidelines.

Reviewing a body of evidence is challenging due to the growing volume of research, variability in study designs, and haphazard and biased access to research. To this end, Naude noted that decision makers face challenges in using vast amounts of primary research to enable informed policy development, making SRs and MAs key to the planning and execution of effective policies.

Naude described the multitude of benefits that MAs and SRs provide for the policy development process. When completed correctly, MAs and SRs can increase transparency and objectivity, reduce bias, capture the totality of evidence on a subject, create more precise results, capture

---

[1] https://training.cochrane.org/handbook (accessed January 3, 2024).
[2] Discussions on combining the numerical results of primary studies for a MA are in the second workshop in this series.

the uncertainty of existing findings, and point to the need for additional research on a topic. Again, Naude reiterated the need for strong, consistent methods to ensure proper protocols and sound decision making.

Naude also spoke about the planning of SRs, describing the four pillars of the planning process:

- Gathering the necessary background information;
- Assembling an author team;
- Assembling adequate resources for the SR; and
- Establishing the question that the SR seeks to answer.

Naude provided a thorough explanation of each pillar. When considering the first pillar of background information, Naude noted that it is important to develop an SR that is "fit to the purpose," which she explained as considering the purported use of the SR, the end product to be informed by the guidance produced by the SR, and the target audience. She also explained that SRs are commonly used when there is a "guidance gap"—a lack of sufficient information to create reliable guidance on an issue or a lack of clarity on how existing guidance should be applied.

Speaking on the second pillar of developing the author team, Naude noted the importance of minimizing conflicts of interest in both funding and nonfinancial interests. She said that one should seek to assemble a "dream team" consisting of specialists with expertise in both methods and subject matter. The team should also include the perspectives of key stakeholders and have a project lead with strong project management and relational skills. The authors of the SR, importantly, should not have a vested interest in the findings of the SR. Objectivity is key, Naude reinforced.

The third pillar is having adequate resources to perform the SR and adhering to an established timeline. The third pillar also focuses on "reliability," which includes good data management and quality assurance processes that allow for data replicability and enhanced credibility. Naude noted that transparent reporting and an audit trail for decision making further enhance credibility. She suggested that new software, and more recently the use of artificial intelligence (AI)-enabled programs, can be used to support this process.

The fourth pillar focuses on the development of the question to be answered by the SR. Naude explained that this question guides all future work during the SR process. She spoke of the importance of taking time to clearly frame and develop the question with the entire team, noting that the question might be a problem statement. She said that the question needs to be clear, but it could be either broad or narrow, depending on the purpose of the SR, which stems from the needs of the user and the context of how the SR will be used. To develop the question, Naude stated that the team should begin by considering the aim of the review and then use the PICO or Population, Exposure, Comparator, Outcome (PECO) construct to develop the question. Using this framework can help the team decide what factors are most critical in the development of their research question.

Naude highlighted that a logic model and conceptual framework are key parts of the planning process for SRs. Because nutrition studies are inherently complex and multi-factorial, logic models are useful for unpacking this complexity and refining the question being asked in the review. Logic models can also help guide the review process in general. The PICO construct might be used at three stages of the review process to help guide decision making. For example, the review PICO planned during the protocol stage helps to decide on the inclusion and exclusion criteria for study eligibility. The PICO for synthesis, which is also planned during the protocol stage, helps the researchers determine the planned comparisons, such as intervention and comparator groups, or groupings of outcomes and population subgroups. Finally, the PICO of the included studies, determined during the review stage, considers what was examined in the studies that have been included in the SR and helps the team understand the extent to which data from these studies, and the review overall, are generalizable.

Naude concluded her presentation by noting the necessity of choosing which outcomes are included in an SR and weighting these outcomes by level of importance. She said that this process fundamentally impacts the strength of an SR. Naude noted that nutrition studies often have many variables, and it is common to encounter different ways of measuring the same outcome. When rating the importance of variables, Naude suggested considering what outcomes are of greatest importance to policy makers that will use the review to inform policy and guideline development. Another way to choose outcomes of interest is by understanding their clinical relevance, which can be enhanced by including subject-matter experts on the review team. Naude also urged researchers to be mindful of the conflicts of interest that may arise with industry involvement in research. Finally, she reminded the audience of the inherent complexity of nutrition research and the common finding of a multiplicity of results. Different studies, even those measuring the same inputs or nutrients, may show varying results. For example, a positive effect could be seen from a nutrient in one study, but another study may show no effect, creating difficulty for teams to combine these results. In these cases, the use of experts remains particularly important to the evaluation and analysis processes.

METHODS FOR REDUCING THE RISK OF BIAS IN SYSTEMATIC REVIEWS AND META-ANALYSES

"Doing a meta-analysis is easy. Doing one well is hard." Quoting Ingram Olkin, a former professor of statistics and education at Stanford University, this sentiment was spoken by Hooper during her remarks at the first of three workshops on the use of MAs in nutrition research and policy.

Hooper began her presentation about the methods for reducing the risk of bias in SRs and MAs. She noted that the methods and resources discussed were largely drawn from Cochrane guidance[3] and training[4] materials. Hooper disclosed that while she had not received industry funding during the last decade, she had received funding from a variety of research organizations. She stated that she has been an editor for the Cochrane Heart Group and Oral Health Group and noted that she is a member of the World Health Organization (WHO) Nutrition Guidance Expert Advisory Group (NUGAG).

Hooper introduced the seven methodological pillars for reducing risk of bias in SRs. They include:

- Writing the protocol;
- Searching for studies;
- Selecting studies and collecting data;
- Assessing risk of bias of included studies;
- Analyzing the data;
- Interpreting the findings; and
- Reporting the review.

Hooper began by describing the second pillar, searching for studies. She said that it is the foundation of a good SR, explaining that searches should span across years, databases, languages, and paradigms. Too narrow a search can add bias, as can a search that only includes research published in English or does not include searches of trials registers. She suggested the importance of working with an expert in developing sensitive and specific search strategies (including searching in "gray" literature, which may include unpublished work, theses, and government papers) to ensure important studies are not missed in this key stage. Hooper stated that the search process should be peer reviewed, detailed, and reproducible. The review

---

[3] For guidance resources, see https://training.cochrane.org/handbook; https://community.cochrane.org/mecir-manual; https://jbi-global-wiki.refined.site/space/MANUAL (all accessed January 3, 2024).

[4] For training resources, see https://training.cochrane.org/interactivelearning; https://www.human.cornell.edu/dns/who-cochrane-cornell-summer-institute (both accessed January 3, 2024).

question (the PICO or PECO formatted question) should inform both the search strategy and the pre-specified criteria for selection of studies.

With respect to the third pillar, selecting studies and collecting data, Hooper suggested that the team consider which papers found in the search fulfill the team's predetermined inclusion criteria and that the assessment of inclusion is done through independent duplication. The research team should refer to the PICO or PECO question and develop rules to resolve disagreements around which studies to include or exclude. Hooper suggested that any disagreements be resolved based on the established inclusion criteria with reference to how the review question is most reliably addressed, and after such a discussion, criteria may be refined (and such refinements reported). The process of assessing inclusion needs to be systematic and recorded in detail.

After studies are selected, data collection occurs. Hooper explained that data collection should be carried out independently in duplicate, and any discrepancies in the data should be discussed within the team. Hooper said that it is important for SRs to gather data on included study methods, participants, interventions, comparators, flow (numbers recruited, dropping out, analyzed) and outcomes. Nutrition reviews also need to collect data on baseline nutrition status and how fully the nutrition intervention was implemented (what exactly was the intervention and how well did the participants stick to it, and the equivalent for observational studies if these are included). She emphasized that outcome data are not monolithic and suggested reaching out to a study's authors when any data outcomes are unclear or presented in a way that cannot be compared with that of other studies, urging vigilance when data do not seem believable. She further stated that rejecting fraudulent data is very important as such data can add extreme bias to an SR.

Hooper addressed several questions that were provided by the workshop sponsor prior to the workshop about best practices for identifying and avoiding extraction errors and miscalculations in mean differences and confidence intervals from the primary studies included in an MA. Hooper stated that when conducting an SR, the key stages are data collection being conducted independently in duplicate with disagreements discussed as a team, pre-specifying data to collect using a trialed data collection sheet and contacting primary study authors to clarify outcome data (and methodological details) when required. In response to the sponsor questions about how to evaluate the quality of an MA when data extraction errors or data errors in the primary studies are found to be present and whether there is a level of error that invalidates the conclusion of an MA, Hooper stated firmly that errors in data should be considered a "red flag" and any SR or MA with data errors should be avoided. Errors in the data and methodology call into question the methodological rigor, value, and validity of the entire SR, she explained.

Hooper detailed some tools that may be useful during the data collection and study selection phases of conducting SRs. Covidence is a tool that enables the independent duplication of assessment of inclusion criteria, data extraction, and risk of bias assessment and allows for remote collaboration with teams around the globe.[5] Hooper explained that much of the review process can be conducted within Covidence, and she stated her opinion that it is an essential tool for a successful review.

Hooper also discussed Rayyan,[6] an AI tool that enables collaborative reviews conducted across a broad research platform and easily allows researchers to independently assess the data in duplication, but it does not allow data extraction and risk of bias assessment to the extent that Covidence does. But it is useful and, importantly, free of charge. Another tool, EPPI Reviewer,[7] supports a range of reviews, including meta-ethnography. Hooper also suggested the use of PlotDigitizer and Microsoft Paint, which can obtain numbers from a visual plot. Hooper noted that these tools enable teams to assess the quality of the evidence to be reviewed as clearly as possible without adding additional bias.

On the topic of the fourth pillar, assessing risk of bias, Hooper noted that bias is an inherent part of all studies. What is critical, she said, is understanding what the bias is, the level of bias, and where the risks of bias may be greatest in each study; the goal cannot be to avoid bias entirely, but to identify, expose, and clarify the bias, helping the author and readers of the SR to understand to what degree the review "answer" is likely to deviate from the true answer to the SR question. Hooper referenced the saying "garbage in, garbage out," explaining that the risk of bias present in a review is a key factor in assessing the quality and relevance of the review. It is important to realize that an MA of biased studies can lead to a precise estimate of the wrong answer. To this end, Hooper offered some methods for avoiding and addressing bias in the review process. First, she said that teams should aim to exclude studies during the screening stage that are believed to have a high risk for bias, such as non-randomized studies. Once studies have been included, she suggested that teams tabulate and report the risk of bias in all included studies (ideally presenting risk of bias for all studies across all domains of bias, and also as part of any forest plot). As part of this process, Hooper suggested that teams run sensitivity analyses within the MA, including all relevant studies in the main analysis, then removing studies at highest risk of bias (such sensitivity analyses should be pre-specified in

---

[5] https://www.covidence.org/ (accessed January 3, 2024).
[6] https://www.rayyan.ai/ (accessed January 3, 2024).
[7] https://eppi.ioe.ac.uk/cms/Default.aspx?tabid=2914 (accessed January 3, 2024).

the review protocol). If sensitivity analysis results differ markedly from the main analysis, Hooper stated, then bias should be suspected and reported. Throughout this process, Hooper suggested using tools such as GRADE to assess, analyze, and present findings on the reliability of the review findings (including bias) for each review outcome. She detailed some unique forms of bias that may be present in observational nutrition studies. For example, dietary exposures are often accompanied by numerous confounders such as socioeconomic status, physical activity levels, or smoking status. Hooper reviewed the risks of bias and study limitations of observational studies, based on information from the GRADE handbook (see Table 2-1).

Hooper also shared some benefits of using cohort studies, such as the potential for a longer follow-up period, the potential to assess a broader set of outcomes, and larger sample sizes than randomized controlled trials (RCTs), making it potentially easier to observe population health effects. Hooper said that both RCTs and cohort studies have their own unique strengths and weaknesses, and it is important to consider the differences between the study types when deciding whether and how to include them in a review. Ideally, if observational studies are systematically reviewed, RCTs should also be searched for and included.

TABLE 2-1 Limitations in Observational Studies

Limitations	Explanation
Failure to develop and apply appropriate eligibility criteria (inclusion of control population)	• Under- or over-matching in case-control studies • Selection of exposed and unexposed in cohort studies from different populations
Flawed measurement of both exposure and outcome	• Differences in measurement of exposure (e.g., recall bias in case-control studies) • Differential surveillance for outcome in exposed and unexposed in cohort studies
Failure to adequately control confounding	• Failure of accurate measurement of all known prognostic factors • Failure to match for prognostic factors and/or adjustment in statistical analysis
Incomplete or inadequately short follow-up	Especially within prospective cohort studies, both groups should be followed for the same amount of time

SOURCES: Presented by Lee Hooper on September 19, 2023, at the workshop on Use of Meta-Analyses in Nutrition Research and Policy: Planning of Meta-Analysis (Schunemann et al., 2013).

Addressing an additional question of how to consider risk of bias when evaluating diet and disease relationships, Hooper suggested that teams assess the risk of bias, report the risk, and use a sensitivity analysis to see if their results change when removing the data considered to be at highest risk for bias.

Hooper spoke about the role of unpublished studies in creating bias in the literature. SRs of observational studies have much greater problems with selective reporting and publication bias than SRs of RCTs as observational studies are less likely to be published than trials if they do not show "statistically significant" effects—so that the published set of studies is unlikely to be representative of the true evidence base. It is easier to identify unpublished and "negative" or "neutral" RCTs than other types of unpublished studies, as RCTs are required to register in advance of being conducted and thus are discoverable through searching of trials registers. Trials registers also provide pre-specified study methods for both published and unpublished studies, allowing research teams to check whether published studies include all planned outcomes, analytical methods, subgroup analyses, etc. The ability to screen for these factors in RCTs enables better assessment of risk of bias for individual trials within the SR, and ultimately for the SR itself. However, Hooper explained that a similar process is not available for identifying unpublished cohort studies or the pre-specified methods of published observational studies. Often only positive associations are published, and negative or non-existent associations may remain unpublished (and so excluded from the SR). Additionally, significant associations may be manufactured by selective subgroup assessments or altered analytical methods. She emphasized that it is critical to analyze the study methods, registry entries, and protocols in every study being considered for inclusion in a review.

Hooper spoke to the question of best practices for addressing publication bias, stating the importance of identifying, acknowledging, and addressing the studies that are missing from the published literature. Hooper emphasized the importance of qualifying SR results by noting the degree to which information may be missing; this is part of the GRADE process.

Hooper addressed pillar five, analyzing the data, and discussed the importance of the protocol that guides the analysis process. She noted that teams should specify in the protocol what effect size is clinically relevant to the research topic and explain the methods of data analysis. Teams should prespecify the comparisons to be made, the effect measures, and all data analysis questions. The protocol should also prespecify methods of data analysis including comparisons to be made, how heterogeneity will be assessed, and what subgroup analyses and sensitivity analyses will be run.

Addressing the question of what criteria should be used to determine whether individual nutrition studies have too many clinical or methodological differences to be combined within the same MA, Hooper responded that teams should only include studies that truly answer the research question and should not combine data from studies that used different methodologies (e.g., differences in treatment, dose, population characteristics, duration, comparators, or diets). She noted that researchers can use subgroupings to answer sub-questions.

Addressing another question about best practices for planning appropriate subgroup analyses and sensitivity analysis a priori, she provided an example using the nutrient selenium. Hooper said to set up the main question and sub-questions, and in this example, the main question might be: "What is the effect of increasing selenium on cognition?" Sub-questions might include, "Does this effect differ by baseline selenium status? Does it differ by baseline cognitive status? Does the effect differ depending on the source of selenium?" To address these sub-questions one would plan meta-analytic subgroups based on baseline selenium status, baseline cognitive status, and selenium source. These subgroups should be integrated into the whole review process, included from the beginning of the review, and relevant information to assess to which subgroup each study belongs should be collected during the main data collection process.

Hooper addressed best practices for interpretation of findings, the sixth of the seven pillars. She stated that interpretation of the results is often the most difficult task, because information is almost always incomplete. She reiterated the importance of using the GRADE tool to assess the certainty of evidence for each outcome. She discussed how GRADE can be used to assess specific indicators of the certainty and reliability of evidence. These are risk of bias, inconsistency, imprecision, and indirectness. Hooper provided examples of how to assess each of these domains, basing assessment of risk of bias on the risk of bias assessment for each outcome (including sensitivity analysis results), inconsistency on measures of heterogeneity, imprecision on the 95% confidence interval around data from the relevant meta-analyses, and imprecision on the generalizability of the included participants to those for whom the answer is needed. GRADE works to evaluate certainty in reviews of both trial and observational evidence. When assessing RCTs, GRADE assumes a higher certainty of evidence but downgrades for problems, while when assessing cohort studies GRADE assumes a lower certainty of evidence but can upgrade for strong evidence (e.g., for a strong dose-response relationship).

For the final portion of her presentation, Hooper focused on the process of reporting a review, the last of the seven pillars. She suggested that researchers use the Preferred Reporting Items for Systematic Reviews and

Meta-Analyses (PRISMA)[8] statement to ensure that their SR is reported comprehensively. PRISMA is an evidence-based minimum set of items for reporting an SR or MA that includes a flow diagram of potential studies and a checklist of the key components to be reported.

Hooper addressed the questions of how MAs can be used to evaluate the strength of evidence when different outcomes are reported in different studies and how MAs can be used to evaluate the strength of the totality of evidence. In response, she provided an example from the development of WHO guidance on saturated fat (SF) consumption (WHO, 2023). WHO commissioned an SR that focused on RCTs of at least 2 years duration that assessed the impact of reducing SF intake on a variety of noncommunicable diseases, such as cardiovascular disease and cancer. In parallel WHO commissioned an SR of prospective cohort studies that assessed associations between SF intake and the same health outcomes. It also commissioned an update of an SR and regression analyses of SF intake and lipid outcomes in highly controlled metabolic studies over short periods of time. For each key outcome within each review the evidence was assessed using GRADE. Consistency in results was found across the three reviews, which was seen as strengthening the totality of evidence. Hooper used this example to demonstrate how a team could approach a complex nutrition research question by making use of different types of evidence to produce a single best answer.

Finally, Hooper mentioned that the commissioning of new SRs and MAs for nutrition guidance may not always be necessary. An alternative solution, she said, may be to locate existing robust SRs that address the topic of interest. The Risk of Bias in Systematic Reviews (ROBIS) tool can be used to quantify whether a particular SR is strong enough to be used for the development of dietary guidance (directly or through updating).[9] The target audience for ROBIS is guideline developers and authors of SRs. Robust existing SRs may need to be updated, and it is good practice, she said, to work with the original review team to accomplish this, and potentially to pre-specify new outcomes, subgroups, and/or sensitivity analyses for the review update to provide the most useful data for guideline development.

---

[8] For information on PRISMA, see http://prisma-statement.org/prismastatement/checklist.aspx?AspxAutoDetectCookieSupport=1 (accessed January 3, 2024).

[9] For information on ROBIS, see https://www.bristol.ac.uk/population-health-sciences/projects/robis/robis-tool/ (accessed January 10, 2024).

PANEL DISCUSSION

A panel discussion was convened, moderated by Amanda J. MacFarlane. MacFarlane began by introducing the additional discussants, Sydne Newberry of the RAND Corporation and Christopher Schmid from Brown University School of Public Health, who joined the conversation with Naude and Hooper. MacFarlane facilitated the discussion, inviting comments from the panelists and questions from audience members.

Transparency

Hooper said that making good decisions, being fully transparent, and not adding additional bias during the SR process is challenging but critical. She suggested that SR authors aim to be clear in their process and intentional in attempts to avoid bias. MacFarlane added that maintaining transparency and reporting any challenges can help preserve trust in a study. Hooper highlighted the importance of teamwork and transparency in the GRADE process, where teams work together to assess the relative quality of their assembled evidence. Newberry agreed, further emphasizing the benefits of transparency at every stage of a review, including the planning stage. She stated the importance of this transparency to the quality of the evidence and the need for high-quality evidence in policy development. Newberry said that policy makers who seek to use the evidence to inform policy and guidelines should have a clear understanding of what the evidence suggests and promotes. For this reason, she noted, researchers should clearly plan and report their SRs to make the evidence both understandable and useful.

Planning and Team Development

Newberry said that one of the biggest challenges of SRs and MAs is working with stakeholders to frame research questions in ways that are truly answerable. She referenced comments from Hooper and Naude about the importance of focusing on the clinical significance of outcomes. However, for many outcomes of interest, Newberry said, the clinically important differences are unknown. Given that many nutrition questions have an overwhelming body of literature and studies have finite sample sizes, Newberry suggested that limits on the quantity of primary studies to gather and assess should be established as part of the review protocol development process.

Newberry disagreed with a comment that Hooper had made during her presentation in which she suggested that study searches should include studies published in languages other than English. Newberry expressed concern that seeking studies in other languages could incur additional costs and time delays for translation. However, Hooper responded that online translation tools have become better and more affordable and are sufficient for an initial translation, allowing reviewers to decide whether a study is otherwise appropriate for inclusion. Additionally, Hooper suggested that students serving as research assistants may also be a useful, low-cost option for further translation needs.

As part of the planning process for SRs, Newberry described the benefits of searching for existing SRs on the topic of interest prior to initiating a new study, noting that many nutrition research questions have already been addressed in SRs published in the past 5 years. This process of seeking existing reviews can be included in the planning process, and those intending to conduct a review to inform policy should decide whether these previous reviews can be used. If not, Newberry suggested mining existing reviews for sources or referencing them in the current work. This suggestion echoed Hooper's previous comment about the use of existing SRs if they are of high quality and truly address the guideline's research question.

Schmid contributed to the discussion of proper planning and reinforced that SRs are only as good as the studies they include and the sampling schemes on which they are based. Including more studies does not inherently mean including the right studies or producing a better review. Schmid further contributed to the discussion on research teams and protocols, saying that one could compare the SR process to that of an RCT. Protocols may be revised numerous times as issues arise, but changes should be documented and agreed upon by all team members. Having all experts involved agree to the protocol is crucial to the process. Schmid shared his experience of the struggles that can result from lack of agreement on the protocol, including having to revise work, which slows down the review. He recommended being as explicit as possible with protocols in advance. Hooper added that having teams do a "trial run" before the review begins can improve the overall efficiency of the process. Although this step may seem burdensome, and MacFarlane noted that the process may be iterative, Hooper advocated that it ultimately helps the process run more smoothly by ensuring that everyone on the team can identify and address disagreements up front. Schmid added that addressing questions about eligibility criteria before beginning the review will lead to increased trust in the study results.

Replying to Schmid's comment about the process of assembling and training teams, Naude noted that for researchers with baseline training in nutritional epidemiology, experiential learning is key. People learn best through experience performing reviews, and repetition builds skills. She also noted that SRs do not always provide definitive answers to research questions, but they move researchers closer to understanding the level of confidence in the answer, which can help inform decision making and policy development. Schmid added that SRs are a wonderful teaching tool for those who want to understand how research is conducted and analyzed. He remarked that if more students outside of the research field had exposure to the SR process during their education, the public's general understanding of science might be improved.

While the discussion centered on the topic of creating effective teams and organizing the review process, audience members asked about the process for building the "dream team" for conducting the review. Specifically, they inquired about who should be included and how roles and responsibilities should be divided among team members. Naude replied that different reviews require different approaches. Generally, she said, a team will include a "lead" or project manager and other members with different areas of expertise. For example, topic area expertise is very important for understanding the biological relevance of outcomes. In other phases of the review, teams may rely less on subject-matter experts and more on data expertise and information specialists. Some review teams may delegate the data extraction process for efficiency purposes. There is no one-size-fits-all approach, she said, and finding a system that works requires repetition and experience. However, Naude acknowledged that the bulk of a review will often be completed by two to four people, with additional experts contributing to the process as needed.

Hooper reinforced the benefits of including experts from the beginning of the process, including protocol development. She said that subject-matter experts, statisticians, search specialists, and SR methodological experts should all be involved in the planning process, to ensure that adequate standards are established. Hooper discussed how to address areas of disagreement during a review and suggested that teams work through points of disagreement together, refining their inclusion and exclusion criteria as questions are resolved. She noted the importance of having a method that the entire team understands and reiterated the significance of planning, noting that SRs require clear guidelines and protocols for an effective process.

Assessing and Addressing Bias

Schmid said that teams should be careful to report as much of the data as possible when those data are of high quality. For example, if a team discovers 100 high-quality studies but only reports on 15 of those studies, that report may not produce a high-quality answer. Hooper concurred, noting that trimming study selection down from 100 to 15, as is necessary in the creation of a forest plot, will add bias and uncertainty. Hooper suggested that while it may not be possible to eliminate this type of bias entirely, it is essential to the process that it be acknowledged and reported, discussing the findings and implications of the missing studies.

Schmid stated his opinion that the meaning of the ratings in the GRADE process are not sufficiently discussed or considered. He added that there are new AI and machine learning tools that can be useful for both screening and extracting data, a point on which Hooper concurred. Schmid mentioned that his team at Brown University has developed an SR repository and a program abstractor that use AI and machine learning. He reinforced the need for strong review teams, with experts in every domain involved in the process.

MacFarlane noted that there are many ways to assess and address bias, including through use of risk of bias tools. Numerous tools exist, and it may be difficult for researchers to determine which tool or method is best for their study. Naude suggested using the most recent Cochrane tool, "Risk of Bias 2," for reducing bias in RCTs. Naude explained that when using the Risk of Bias 2 tool, reviewers have the option to change the weighting of different domains. With study designs that are not RCTs, Naude suggested the use of other tools to reduce bias and urged having rules in place a priori to manage overall judgments. Consistent application of methods and tools is key, she reiterated.

Hooper agreed that Risk of Bias 2 is a very useful tool, although she and Naude agreed that it is slightly more difficult to operate than Risk of Bias 1. Hooper added that it is critical to focus on the risk of bias that is most relevant to the specific area of study or the bias that would have the greatest impact on the results of the review. Newberry added that since most nutrition studies are cohort studies, not RCTs, the Risk of Bias in Non-randomized Studies–of Interventions (ROBINS-I) or Risk of Bias in Non-randomized Studies–of Exposures (ROBINS-E) may be useful to assess risk of bias. Newberry also suggested the Newcastle-Ottawa Scale (NOS) tool for assessing quality of non-randomized studies in MAs. However, she noted that these tools may not be sensitive enough to detect all types of bias. Schmid and Hooper suggested conducting a sensitivity analysis, first conducting meta-analysis of all studies, then eliminating studies that have a high risk of bias and running the analysis again to see whether the results change. Schmid and Hooper concluded that when the results change during this process, there may be uncertainty about the usefulness of the results.

MacFarlane posed a question to the panel about how to address the bias that may result from the lack of clear control groups in nutrition studies. For example, she explained, drug trials often have clear treatment and placebo groups, but nutrition interventions may rely on baseline nutrition status as a control group. She noted that this can cause challenges given that baseline nutrition status can be an imprecise and poorly reported measurement. Naude replied, stating that research teams should look for nuance in the study design of the included studies to understand whether their question or intervention has been altered to accommodate the imprecision of baseline nutrition status as a control group. She also said that subgroup analyses can be difficult to conduct in this context. Naude added that this challenge emphasizes the need to improve reporting of the primary research and ensure that every study included meets basic reporting guidelines. Poor, inadequate, and vague reporting in primary studies will negatively impact the review process and outcomes. Naude noted that this highlights the importance of having established methods and applying tools consistently to avoid imprecision and bias.

In closing, Naude said that the key to addressing problems in SRs and MAs is to continue to highlight and discuss them. She also noted that developments in technology promise advancements in the field in general, and improvements to data collection, organization, and analysis.

3

Exploring Best Practices of Conducting Meta-Analysis

This chapter describes the presentations and discussions that took place during the second workshop, titled Use of Meta-Analyses in Nutrition Research and Policy: Exploring Best Practices of Conducting Meta-Analysis, which took place on September 25, 2023. The objectives of the workshop were to

- Explore best practices for screening data for potential errors;
- Discuss a system for evaluation of risk of bias of study design;
- Discuss a system for evaluation of study results, including precision and consistency of estimates and the potential for publication bias; and
- Explain how to interpret the results of meta-analyses (MAs), what to do if assumptions are violated, and whether it is expected to have higher statistical heterogeneity for nutrition studies.

The workshop was moderated by planning committee member Janet A. Tooze from Wake Forest University and included presentations by Emma Boyland of the University of Liverpool, Andrew Jones of Liverpool John Moores University, and George A. Wells of the University of Ottawa. A panel discussion with the three presenters and additional discussants Elie A. Akl of the American University of Beirut, Joseph Beyene of McMaster University, and M. Hassan Murad of the Mayo Clinic followed the presentations. The workshop concluded with remarks from planning committee member Russell Jude de Souza of McMaster University. Workshop speakers addressed the following questions, which were provided by the workshop sponsor in advance of the workshop:

- Extraction errors from the primary studies included in MAs are common. What are best practices for avoiding/identifying these types of errors?
- What are the best practices for addressing publication bias?

BEST PRACTICES OF META-ANALYSIS IN NUTRITION RESEARCH

Boyland's, Jones's, and Wells's presentations on best practices of MA in nutrition research covered four topic areas:

- Screening data for potential data errors;
- Evaluating risk of bias of study design;
- Evaluating study results, including precision and consistency of estimates and the potential for publication bias; and
- Interpreting the results of MA, including statistical heterogeneity.

Screening Data for Extraction Errors

Boyland began by focusing on screening data for potential extraction errors. She disclosed that she receives no industry funding and approached the presentation through the lens of an academic researcher, leaning on her experience as a lead reviewer for the World Health Organization (WHO). Her presentation drew content from reviews that she cocreated with other experts. Finally, Boyland noted that her presentation included information from the Cochrane Handbook, which she highlighted as a key resource for anyone conducting an MA.

Boyland stated that the best practice should be to prevent data errors from occurring during data extraction and highlighted the importance of training. For example, Boyland emphasized the importance of training the entire research team on all aspects of the process, including consistent methods of data extraction and she endorsed the careful examination of retraction statements to ensure that none of the data being extracted for inclusion has been retracted. She echoed the sentiments of Hooper, recommending that data extraction occur independently and in duplicate. She noted that this duplication is particularly important for any data elements that require subjective judgments and for data that are integral to the outcomes of the MA being performed.

Boyland suggested cross-checking all presentations of the data, including tables, text, and figures, for accuracy and homogeneity. She also noted the benefits of a standardized data extraction template table, which can improve data organization and prevent errors in extraction and presentation of the data. An example of a data extraction template table is provided in Figure 3-1. Boyland described the "balancing act" between extracting too much and too little data. She recommended that teams consider the data and figures they intend to present in their review when determining the data to extract.

Boyland discussed the potential complication of duplicate data, or "linked data or studies," which occurs when multiple papers are based on the same data set. She emphasized the importance of screening for linked data to avoid including duplicate data within an MA, noting that it may not be obvious that data are linked. She highlighted some factors to screen for, including identical locations, sample sizes, study dates, and study durations. If it is not clear whether two studies shared the same data, Boyland suggested reaching out to the study authors to verify. She referenced her own experience with this situation, discussing a time in which her team was performing an MA and encountered two articles that did not mention being connected but had similar characteristics. One was titled "Food advertising, children's food choices and obesity: interplay of cognitive defenses and product evaluation: an experimental study" (Tarabashkina et al., 2016). The second article was called "When persuasive intent and product's healthiness make a difference for young consumers" (Tarabashkina et al., 2018). The authors were similar and the data in general appeared similar, although not identical. Boyland's team contacted the study authors, who confirmed that the data were linked. At this point, the team relied on pre-specified decision rules to determine which study to include in the MA, to avoid including duplicate data.

In cases where two or more papers with linked data are discovered, the team must decide which paper to include in their MA. Boyland suggested having a decision-making protocol for this specific issue included in the initial protocol for the MA so that the decision-making process is formal and systematic. For example, she said that teams might agree in advance to always use the more recently published article. She emphasized that it is critical for the review authors to choose which paper to include and to provide justification for this decision.

Other situations that can cause confusion in the data extraction process are instances when data from two studies are reported within the same article. Boyland gave some examples of this problem, such as two similar studies being reported in one paper, two randomized controlled trials (RCTs) with the same study design being carried out separately with male and female participants, or two RCTs performed identically but in different countries. She explained that it is not necessary to exclude these types of papers from the MA, but it is important that the data extraction and

Data extraction	Methods	Participants	Intervention	Outcomes	Results
• Date • Initials of extractor • Article identifier	• Design • Randomization • Statistical analysis • Funding/COI	• Setting • Country • Eligibility criteria • Characteristics (e.g., age, sex)	• Intervention(s) and comparator(s) • Components: dose, timing, duration, frequency	• For each domain (e.g., intake) • Measurement tool • Metric • Aggregation • Timing	• N/% included • Summary (e.g., mean ± SD) • Estimates and precision (e.g., odds ratio, 95% CI)

FIGURE 3-1 An example of a data extraction template.

NOTE: CI = confidence interval; COI = conflict of interest; SD = standard deviation.

SOURCE: Presented by Emma Boyland on September 25, 2023, at the workshop on Use of Meta-Analyses in Nutrition Research and Policy: Best Practices of Conducting Meta-Analysis.

analysis clearly note that the two data sets came from the same article. For example, she offered an option of listing the data by study author, then year, and then noting either "study 1" or "study 2."

Another place where errors can arise is when multiple outcomes are reported within the same study. Boyland said that this may occur when there are different data points within the same article that seem relevant to the data being extracted. She gave the example of an MA on media usage. One article may report on both time spent viewing television and time spent online, and the team needs to decide which data to extract. Boyland suggested referring to the pre-established protocol in the decision-making process, asking which data are most relevant to the MA, and which data sets use the most valid tools. She illustrated this point with another example from the food marketing literature, noting that when examining the effects of exposure to food marketing on participant food intake, there are many different but potentially relevant outcomes. The team involved in this example decided to consider the most relevant outcomes to the purpose of their specific review, which, in this case, was the reduction of unhealthy food intake. In the absence of this outcome, they had a secondary outcome, which was total energy-dense snack intake. Having these criteria and outcomes established in advance enabled the team to make consistent, uniform decisions throughout the review process.

Evaluation of Risk of Bias in Study Design

In the second portion of her presentation, Boyland discussed the evaluation of risk of bias in study design. This type of bias, she explained, refers to "systematic errors" or deviation from the truth in results. This form of error is distinct from random errors or imprecision, and it may be introduced into the data at many points throughout the research process, including from the original article authors through research design constraints or by systematic review (SR) authors. She detailed some of the ways that systematic errors may occur. For example, study authors may have bias that is reflected in the selective reporting of results. Review authors can additionally add their own bias in how they select studies and report data. Research constraints can impact the quality of results by causing researchers to rely on less precise data—for example, some studies rely on self-reported body weight as the only measurement of weight. Importantly, Boyland noted that it is important to consciously minimize bias wherever possible. As stated previously, this bias can come from the primary studies, research constraints, or the SR authors, and she highlighted that bias can either inflate or underestimate an effect.

Boyland described specific tools that can be used to analyze the risk of bias in a study when selecting studies for a review. She explained that the tools should be selected based on their suitability for the specific study design being assessed. For example, as mentioned in Chapter 2, the Cochrane Risk of Bias 2 tool is a highly effective tool when analyzing RCTs for bias.[1] It highlights ways that bias can arise, including during the randomization process, when deviating from the intended intervention, when outcome data are missing, from the way an outcome is measured, and in selecting the data to be reported. She added that each of these domains has an algorithm underlying the tool and explained how studies are rated within this tool. Boyland said that studies can be rated low risk, some concern, or high risk. The tool generates a table depicting the ratings for each domain as well as an overall rating for each article included. Boyland made specific note that "low risk" in one domain does not mean that an entire study is at a low risk for bias and concern in any domain suggests concern with the entire article.

Boyland gave some examples of assessing risk of bias in nutrition research specifically. She highlighted themes from Chapter 2, noting that many of the tools used for analyzing risk of bias are only applicable to RCTs. It is important to consider that many nutrition studies are not RCTs but rather observational studies, necessitating other types of bias assessment tools. As she closed her presentation, Boyland listed some of the most common quality and bias issues that can arise within nutrition research. She noted that nutrition studies, when experimental, often involve small populations measured over short periods of time. She suggested that nutrition research can have a higher overall risk of bias profile than other types of research due to lack of disclosures or bias not being adequately reported in the initial article. She highlighted the common issue of research constraints, pointing out that it is nearly impossible to have a "blinded" experimental group in a nutrition trial. Boyland reiterated that many of the existing tools for examining risk of bias do not apply to the type of studies generally conducted in the nutrition field, and while new tools may need to be created to solve this issue, the creation of new tools can itself lead to errors, if not fully validated.

Addressing Publication Bias

Jones's presentation focused on best practices for avoiding and addressing publication bias in SRs and MAs. Jones disclosed that he would reference work created alongside other researchers as well as materials from the Cochrane Handbook. He defined publication bias as the "failure to publish the results of a study on the basis of the direction or strength of the study findings," a problem not limited to the field of nutrition (DeVito and

---

[1] https://methods.cochrane.org/bias/resources/rob-2-revised-cochrane-risk-bias-tool-randomized-trials (accessed January 10, 2024).

Goldacre, 2019). As he explained, journals are more likely to publish studies that report significant results. He referred to this issue as "file drawer bias" because many studies that do not produce the intended results remain unpublished, or in the "file drawer." He noted that this problem not only occurs when studies have nonsignificant results but also can occur when studies that produce negative results are suppressed by the study sponsor. He expanded on this point, saying that negative findings are generally published more slowly than positive findings, and publication bias is not limited to the field of nutrition. In general, there is a "constrained evidence base" of positive findings. He referenced a study from Polanin et al. (2016), which showed that published studies yield larger effect sizes than unpublished studies.

Jones noted that the prevalence of assessing publication bias is also high. A study titled "Publication Bias in Psychological Science: Prevalence, Methods for Identifying and Controlling, and Implications for the Use of Meta-Analyses" (Ferguson and Brannick, 2012) showed that across 91 MAs, 70 percent demonstrated some effort to evaluate publication bias, and 41 percent reported some evidence of publication bias. He said that it was important to identify unpublished studies, and he described several resources, including preprint servers such as "Nutri-Xiv" for nutrition research. He noted some issues, however, that may arise when using unpublished research. First, the studies are often not peer reviewed. Unpublished studies are more likely to include grammatical and numerical errors as well as errors in their figures and are also less likely than their peer-reviewed counterparts to report conflicts of interest or funding sources, both of which are critical for evaluating overall bias. Despite these challenges, Jones explained that the Preferred Reporting Items for Systematic Reviews and Meta-Analyses (PRISMA) still recommends the use of preprints in MAs to avoid publication bias.

Jones described several statistical methods to assess publication bias. He suggested not using the fail-safe N (FSN) to avoid publication bias. FSN determines the number of studies with a nonsignificant effect that would need to be added to a sample of studies for the meta-analytic effect to be nonsignificant. The focus of this method rests on effect significance rather than effect size. This method is discouraged in nutrition research MAs because it does not actually determine whether there is bias, and the existence of greater bias can lead to the creation of a larger FSN value. For these reasons, Jones noted, the method is not recommended by Cochrane.

Funnel plots, however, can be a useful way to visually examine and identify publication bias. Jones displayed a funnel plot diagram, as shown in Figure 3-2, and described how it can be used to identify publication bias. As he explained, high-powered studies appear at the top of the funnel and lower-powered studies at the bottom. The funnel plot shows each study's

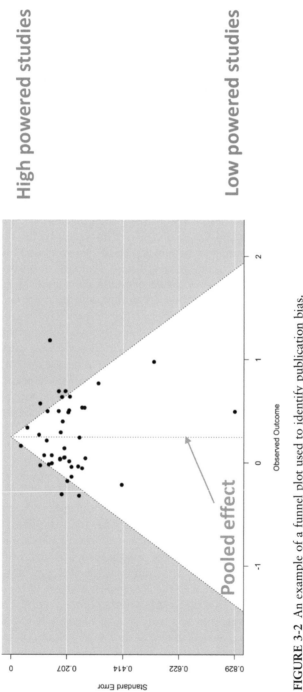

FIGURE 3-2 An example of a funnel plot used to identify publication bias.
SOURCE: Presented by Andrew Jones on September 25, 2023, at the workshop on Use of Meta-Analyses in Nutrition Research and Policy: Best Practices of Conducting Meta-Analysis.

effect size, or intervention effect, against a measure of the study's precision, such as sample size or standard error. Symmetry in the funnel plot suggests a lower risk of publication bias. However, Jones noted, funnel plots are subjective measures, and he referenced a study by Terrin et al. (2005) in which researchers were unable to accurately identify publication bias using visual analysis of a funnel plot. He stated that funnel plots can be difficult to visually interpret when the sample size is small. Jones explained that the improper or misleading use of funnel plots can be harmful and should be used in conjunction with another statistical method.

Jones spoke about methods of assessing funnel plots using statistical analyses. Egger's test aims to identify whether there may be "small study bias" and regresses the scaled effect size against the precision of the included studies. If there is asymmetry this indicates that the smaller studies are systematically different from the larger studies. Another set of tests, the Precision Effect Test (PET) or the Precision Effect Estimate with Standard Error (PEESE) test, fits a linear regression line and then extrapolates to estimate the effect size of a hypothetical study with a standard error of zero. Jones cautioned that this method can be particularly ineffective under conditions of high heterogeneity and when analyzing smaller studies with a large effect size.

Another approach for analyzing a funnel plot that Jones described is the "Trim and Fill" method. In this process, studies with the most extreme effect sizes are "trimmed" from the plot to help researchers understand how many hypothetical studies are missing from the analysis in order to achieve symmetry on the plot. However, he noted some drawbacks to this approach, including that removing outliers will have a large impact and the approach does not work in MAs with high heterogeneity.

Jones also spoke about a method called the p-curve analysis. Jones explained that p-curve analysis is a newer method and for this reason is not frequently used. He described the p-curve analysis as an MA of the p-values in the included studies, and he explained that this is a method of considering the evidential value of the studies being analyzed. Jones said that it is a useful way of measuring publication bias or "selective reporting." He explained that scientists often use the p-value as a measure of importance, and a p-value of less than .05 is used as a threshold for statistical significance in a study but also represents a threshold at which studies are more likely to be published. P-values closer to .01 suggest high-quality evidence with greater power and stronger evidence of effect. When using p-curve analysis, selective reporting may be suspected if p-values cluster around .04 or .05, suggesting that researchers may have engaged in selective reporting of evidence to support their preformed conclusions. He and Boyland used this technique in their MA "Association of Food and Nonalcoholic Beverage Marketing with Children and Adolescents' Eating Behaviors and Health"

(Boyland et al., 2022). In this study, the researchers found strong evidence for the value of the data with more p-values around .01 than .05.

Another method of analysis that Jones touched on is the Graphical Display of Study Heterogeneity (GOSH). This tool can be used to identify the impact of influential studies within an MA (Olkin et al., 2012). It takes the effect size from each study included in the MA and calculates an estimated overall effect for every potential combination of effect size up to a specified number of potential combinations. For an MA of k ≥ 2 studies, where k is the number of studies included in the MA, there are $2^k -1$ potential subsets of studies. For an MA with 20 studies, he noted that there are more than 1 million possible combinations. The purpose of this method of analysis is to gain an understanding of the normal distribution of possible effects from the studies included in the MA. As shown in Figure 3-3, Jones noted that smaller or more heterogeneous MAs will not show a normal distribution curve, and one study with a large effect can bias all the models in which it is included.

In closing, Jones reiterated the importance of checking for unpublished research on the topic being reviewed and using statistical tests to check for publication bias. Examination of the inclusion of influential studies can improve understanding of how they may impact measures of heterogeneity and skew the meta-analytic effect. While each statistical test that he mentioned has both benefits and weaknesses, when more tests are applied, research teams will be better able to demonstrate that their data are sensitive to the potential for publication bias.

INTERPRETING THE RESULTS OF META-ANALYSES AND ADDRESSING HETEROGENEITY

Wells presented on the topics of interpreting the results of MA and how to conceptualize and address heterogeneity. He disclosed that he has no industry funding and stated that he is affiliated with Cochrane, having been a part of the working group since its inaugural meeting. Wells's presentation was informed by his experience with both Cochrane and Grading of Recommendations Assessment, Development and Evaluation (GRADE). The presentation focused on the final three steps in performing an MA:

- Combining the results of selected studies to obtain a summary effect;
- Exploring the differences between the studies, or heterogeneity; and
- Interpreting the results.

Wells described several statistical methods used in these processes. Forest plots are a graphical display of all the individual estimated results

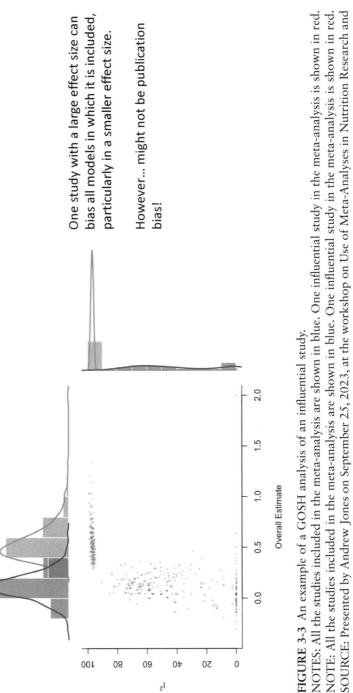

One study with a large effect size can bias all models in which it is included, particularly in a smaller effect size.

However... might not be publication bias!

FIGURE 3-3 An example of a GOSH analysis of an influential study.
NOTES: All the studies included in the meta-analysis are shown in blue. One influential study in the meta-analysis is shown in red.
NOTE: All the studies included in the meta-analysis are shown in blue. One influential study in the meta-analysis is shown in red.
SOURCE: Presented by Andrew Jones on September 25, 2023, at the workshop on Use of Meta-Analyses in Nutrition Research and Policy: Best Practices of Conducting Meta-Analysis.

from scientific studies addressing the same question, along with the overall results. Wells discussed how to use a forest plot to analyze the effect estimates or, in the specific example he reviewed, the "mean difference" data. As Wells described, Figure 3-4 displays a forest plot for the SR on the use of low-sodium salt substitutes (LSSS) compared with regular salt or no active intervention in adults and change in blood pressure. Wells described how to interpret the mean difference information. The horizontal line represents the confidence interval (CI), the vertical line indicates the line of no effect, and if the 95 percent confidence interval crosses the vertical line, it indicates that the results of the study were not statistically significant. Wells also described how the studies were weighted to assess their impact within the MA.

Wells also described two statistical models of analysis that are used in MAs, the equations for which are shown in Figure 3-5: the fixed effects model and the random effects model. The fixed effects model, Wells said, may be unrealistic to use in nutrition MAs because it ignores heterogeneity. The random effects model allows for incorporation of between studies heterogeneity but still requires an understanding of the estimate of the distribution of studies. This estimated distribution may not be accurate if there are few studies or events.

Wells described the "mean difference," an effect measure for comparing the effect means of the intervention groups to those of the control groups. He spoke about how confidence intervals relate to the mean difference, pooling estimates, and standard errors. He said that there should be a lower confidence interval and an upper confidence interval; the more precise the numerical estimates are, the narrower the confidence interval will be. Wells said that the pooled effect estimate is represented both graphically and numerically. Graphically, it is represented on the forest plot by a diamond shaped mark, which highlights its position relative to the mean difference. The numeric value of the pooled estimate effect shows its meta-analytic value, while the confidence interval, and where it falls relative to the individual studies, shows its statistical significance.

Wells discussed how to identify heterogeneity on a forest plot visually, using a chi-square (or Q) test, or by using an I-squared statistical test. Confidence intervals that show very little overlap on the forest plot provide an early indicator of a heterogeneity problem. Even confidence intervals that fall on the same side of the line can be too scattered to overlap and can cause an issue with heterogeneity, he explained. This visual representation is the most basic way to identify excessive heterogeneity. When using the Q-test to assess heterogeneity, a small p-value means that the presence of homogeneity has been rejected and the studies are too different to combine. However, the Q-test as a statistical method can be unreliable with a small body of studies and can also be unreliable with too large of a body of studies due to its high sensitivity. Another issue with the Q-test is that it

Analysis 1.1. Comparison 1: Low-sodium salt substitutes versus regular salt or no active intervention in adults, Outcome 1: Change in DBP (mmHg)

Study or Subgroup	MD	SE	LSSS intervention Total	Control Total	Weight	Mean Difference IV, Random, 95% CI	Mean Difference IV, Random, 95% CI	Risk of Bias A B C D E F G H I J K L M
Allaert 2013 (1)	-4.2	2.36614	21	19	3.2%	-4.20 [-8.84, 0.44]		
Allaert 2017 (2)	-7.4	1.987451	22	19	3.9%	-7.40 [-11.30, -3.50]		
Geleijnse 1994 (3)	-4.1	0.236746	48	49	7.8%	-4.10 [-4.56, -3.64]		
Gilleran 1996 (4)	-1.7	3.8113	11	8	1.6%	-1.70 [-9.17, 5.77]		
Hu 2018 (5)	-0.17	0.341016	243	259	7.7%	-0.17 [-0.84, 0.50]		
Li 2014 (6)	-1.3	0.813878	198	205	7.3%	-1.30 [-2.90, 0.30]		
Li 2016 (7)	0	0.55077	1293	1272	7.3%	0.00 [-1.08, 1.08]		
Mu 2003 (8)	-3.5	2.088178	88	97	3.7%	-3.50 [-7.59, 0.59]		
Neal 2021 (9)	-0.8	0.459154	7436	7081	7.5%	-0.80 [-1.70, 0.10]		
Omvik 1995 (10)	-3.2	3.0103	19	20	2.3%	-3.20 [-9.10, 2.70]		
Pereira 2005 (11)	-4.9	3.557109	12	10	1.8%	-4.90 [-11.87, 2.07]		
Sarikkinen 2011 (1)	-4	2.028073	22	23	3.8%	-4.00 [-7.97, -0.03]		
Suppa 1988 (12)	-2	1.026733	163	159	6.2%	-2.00 [-4.01, 0.01]		
Toft 2020 (13)	-0.116	1.371969	41	49	5.3%	-0.12 [-2.81, 2.57]		
Yu 2021 (14)	-1.2	0.503822	242	234	7.4%	-1.20 [-2.19, -0.21]		
Zhang 2015 (15)	-1.6	1.04338	279	218	6.1%	-1.60 [-3.64, 0.44]		
Zhao 2014 (14)	-3	1.336061	141	141	5.4%	-3.00 [-5.62, -0.38]		
Zhou 2009 (16)	-4.8	1.0459	119	129	6.1%	-4.80 [-6.85, -2.75]		
Zhou 2013 (17)	-4.62	1.043047	213	227	6.1%	-4.62 [-6.66, -2.58]		
Total (95% CI)			**10611**	**10219**	**100.0%**	**-2.43 [-3.50, -1.36]**		

Heterogeneity: Tau² = 3.77; Chi² = 154.08, df = 18 (P < 0.00001); I² = 88%
Test for overall effect: Z = 4.45 (P < 0.00001)
Test for subgroup differences: Not applicable

Favours LSSS intervention   Favours regular salt

FIGURE 3-4 Forest plot for a systematic review of low-sodium salt substitutes and diastolic blood pressure.
SOURCES: Presented by George A. Wells on September 25, 2023, at the workshop on Use of Meta-Analyses in Nutrition Research and Policy: Best Practices of Conducting Meta-Analysis (Brand et al., 2022).

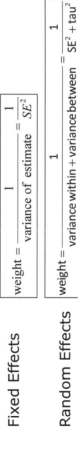

Fixed Effects

$$\text{weight} = \frac{1}{\text{variance of estimate}} = \frac{1}{SE^2}$$

Random Effects

$$\text{weight} = \frac{1}{\text{variance within} + \text{variance between}} = \frac{1}{SE^2 + tau^2}$$

$$\text{pooled estimate} = \frac{\text{sum of (estimate} \times \text{weight)}}{\text{sum of weights}}$$

FIGURE 3-5 Equations used in the fixed effects and random effects models.
SOURCE: Presented by George A. Wells on September 25, 2023, at the workshop on Use of Meta-Analyses in Nutrition Research and Policy: Best Practices of Conducting Meta-Analysis.

lacks nuance and can only produce a "yes or no" answer about the presence of heterogeneity. Another statistical method for assessing the presence of heterogeneity that Wells detailed is the I-squared test, which attempts to identify and quantify heterogeneity. Values range from zero to 100 percent, with higher values indicating higher heterogeneity. While the I-squared test provides more detailed information about the presence of heterogeneity, there is no universally accepted cut-off point for interpretation. For example, below 30–40 percent might represent low or unimportant heterogeneity, 30–60 percent might represent moderate heterogeneity, 50–90 percent might represent substantial heterogeneity, and 75–100 percent might represent high heterogeneity, but these are not firm or specific metrics.

Wells said that once heterogeneity is identified, it should be explained; if it cannot be explained, the data should be interpreted to accommodate the heterogeneity. Wells defined the types of heterogeneity that may be present in an SR or MA. Clinical heterogeneity refers to differences in studies among participant and intervention characteristics. Participant variations may include differences in their condition, demographics, or location. Intervention variations may include differences in implementation, the experience of practitioners involved, and the type of control used, such as placebo, standard care, or no control. Outcomes variations may include measurement methods, event definition, cut points, and duration of follow-up. Methodological heterogeneity, as Wells described, can arise when studies vary in how they are designed and conducted or when there are publication limitations or constraints. Statistical heterogeneity occurs when the results observed across studies are more disparate than would be expected by chance.

Wells described ways to explore heterogeneity. Subgroup analysis and meta-regression can be used to assess the factors that appear to modify the effect. Wells explained that specific factors should be considered during subgroup analyses, such as whether the heterogeneity found within subgroups differs from the overall heterogeneity. He also suggested conducting statistical tests for subgroup differences to ensure that true differences exist between subgroups. Wells noted that confidence in the results of the MA should increase if the effect that is seen is also thought to be clinically plausible and supported by evidence outside of the review.

He suggested exploring heterogeneity through use of sensitivity analysis, which provides information on the robustness of the results. This analysis is done by repeating the MA using alternative options to assess the consistency or robustness of the results. Using the study on LSSS mentioned previously as an example, Wells described the subgroup analyses performed and their results. As he explained, subgroup analysis was conducted by study duration. The study team further meta-analyzed the subgroups and found that there was a moderate I-squared or a moderate risk of heterogeneity.

He described the concept of considering heterogeneity with subgroups and noted the importance of asking whether the subgroups are truly different.

Wells detailed the system of color-coding for evaluating risk of bias within individual studies. Figure 3-6 provides a chart displaying how studies can be rated on a variety of domains, with green signifying low risk of bias, yellow signifying uncertain risk, and red signifying high risk.

While examining the forest plot for the LSSS studies, Wells referred to Jones's description of a GOSH analysis. Wells suggested that it could be useful to remove each study, one at a time, and rerun a GOSH analysis to determine the impact of each individual study on the overall effect.

Wells provided a detailed example of analyzing risk of bias and heterogeneity in an MA featuring studies with binary or discrete outcomes such as studies of cardiovascular events. He described a forest plot that included five RCTs in an MA. He reviewed each component of the forest plot, again describing all the measurements that are graphically displayed on a forest plot. Wells explained that the effect estimates were different in this example due to the binary nature of the outcomes. Relative risk, he explained, is a more straightforward calculation when analyzing discrete outcomes compared with studies that examine multicomponent interventions and complex outcomes. Wells said that there is greater potential for confounding in nutrition studies compared with placebo-controlled drug trials. In the case of a nutrition study focused on sodium intake and cardiovascular events, a control group could be a group consuming table salt in normal amounts or a group that received no active intervention. Another variable that adds potential heterogeneity is whether participants received education on reducing sodium intake. When it comes to studies on LSSS, multifactorial interventions add complexity to the research, and Wells posited that it may not be possible to truly isolate the LSSS as a causative factor. Referring back to the Population, Intervention, Comparator, Outcome (PICO) framework, Wells said that in nutrition studies, the "P" (population) and the "O" (outcome) are commonly easy to define, but the "I" (intervention) and the "C" (control) can be complicated and challenging to define in a singular manner, thus making them difficult to combine and analyze. These challenges present barriers to conducting high-quality nutrition MAs.

Wells explained how one could use the GRADE approach for assessing the certainty of the evidence in which the intervention and control are complicated and not uniform across studies. When this method was applied to the studies in his example, an overall grade of "uncertain" was given, mostly due to the high levels of heterogeneity across the study methods. These inconsistencies and high heterogeneity could not be explained using subgroup analysis or meta-regression, which led to less certainty in the observed effect. Furthermore, Wells noted that the certainty of evidence was further reduced when it was found that the greatest effect was seen in a

Analysis 1.1. Comparison 1: Low-sodium salt substitutes versus regular salt or no active intervention in adults, Outcome 1: Change in DBP (mmHg)

Study or Subgroup	MD	SE	LSSS intervention Total	Control Total	Weight	Mean Difference IV, Random, 95% CI
Allaert 2013 (1)	-4.2	2.36614	21	19	3.2%	-4.20 [-8.84, 0.44]
Allaert 2017 (2)	-7.4	1.987451	22	19	3.9%	-7.40 [-11.30, -3.50]
Geleijnse 1994 (3)	-4.1	0.236746	48	49	7.8%	-4.10 [-4.56, -3.64]
Gilleran 1996 (4)	-1.7	3.8113	11	8	1.6%	-1.70 [-9.17, 5.77]
Hu 2018 (5)	-0.17	0.341016	243	259	7.7%	-0.17 [-0.84, 0.50]
Li 2014 (6)	-1.3	0.813878	198	205	6.7%	-1.30 [-2.90, 0.30]
Li 2016 (7)	0	0.55077	1293	1272	7.3%	0.00 [-1.08, 1.08]
Mu 2003 (8)	-3.5	2.088178	88	97	3.7%	-3.50 [-7.59, 0.59]
Neal 2021 (9)	-0.8	0.459154	7436	7081	7.5%	-0.80 [-1.70, 0.10]
Omvik 1995 (10)	-3.2	3.0103	19	20	2.3%	-3.20 [-9.10, 2.70]
Pereira 2005 (11)	-4.9	3.557109	12	10	1.8%	-4.90 [-11.87, 2.07]
Sarkkinen 2011 (1)	-4	2.028073	22	23	3.8%	-4.00 [-7.97, -0.03]
Suppa 1988 (12)	-2	1.026733	163	159	6.2%	-2.00 [-4.01, 0.01]
Toft 2020 (13)	-0.116	1.371969	41	49	5.3%	-0.12 [-2.81, 2.57]
Yu 2021 (14)	-1.2	0.503822	242	234	7.4%	-1.20 [-2.19, -0.21]
Zhang 2015 (15)	-1.6	1.04338	279	218	6.1%	-1.60 [-3.64, 0.44]
Zhao 2014 (14)	-3	1.336061	141	141	5.4%	-3.00 [-5.62, -0.38]
Zhou 2009 (16)	-4.8	1.0459	119	129	6.1%	-4.80 [-6.85, -2.75]
Zhou 2013 (17)	-4.62	1.043047	213	227	6.1%	-4.62 [-6.66, -2.58]
Total (95% CI)			10611	10219	100.0%	-2.43 [-3.50, -1.36]

Heterogeneity: Tau² = 3.77; Chi² = 154.08, df = 18 (P < 0.00001); I² = 88%
Test for overall effect: Z = 4.45 (P < 0.00001)
Test for subgroup differences: Not applicable

Favours LSSS intervention / Favours regular salt (-20 -10 0 10 20)

Risk of Bias: A B C D E F G H I J K L M

FIGURE 3-6 An example of rating risk of bias through color coding in a forest plot.
SOURCES: Presented by George A. Wells on September 25, 2023, at the workshop on Use of Meta-Analyses in Nutrition Research and Policy: Best Practices of Conducting Meta-Analysis (Brand et al., 2022).

continued

42

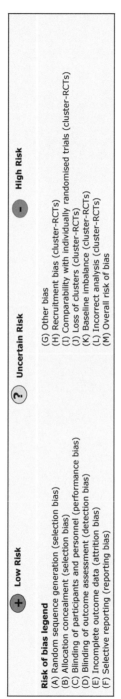

Risk of bias legend
(A) Random sequence generation (selection bias)
(B) Allocation concealment (selection bias)
(C) Blinding of participants and personnel (performance bias)
(D) Blinding of outcome assessment (detection bias)
(E) Incomplete outcome data (attrition bias)
(F) Selective reporting (reporting bias)
(G) Other bias
(H) Recruitment bias (cluster-RCTs)
(I) Comparability with individually randomised trials (cluster-RCTs)
(J) Loss of clusters (cluster-RCTs)
(K) Baseline imbalance (cluster-RCTs)
(L) Incorrect analysis (cluster-RCTs)
(M) Overall risk of bias

+ Low Risk   **?** Uncertain Risk   **−** High Risk

FIGURE 3-6 Continued

study of individuals who were at high risk for cardiovascular events, meaning that this evidence could not be extrapolated to the general population.

Wells described potential reasons for downgrading the certainty of the evidence, including studies that are poorly conducted or inconsistent, study results that do not apply to the question being asked in the MA, small sample sizes, large confidence intervals, and publication bias. Using the MA on the use of LSSS for reducing cardiovascular events as an example, Wells noted that the GRADE method illuminated issues with the quality of evidence, especially for the groups of interest to the MA. Use of this tool helped the researchers to better understand the limitations of the certainty of the evidence.

Wells also suggested the use of A MeaSurement Tool to Assess systematic Reviews (AMSTAR),[2] which he described as a critical appraisal tool for SRs and MAs that include both randomized and non-randomized studies of health care interventions.

PANEL DISCUSSION

The workshop featured a panel discussion with Boyland, Jones, and Wells as well as three additional discussants: Joseph Beyene of McMaster University, Elie A. Akl of the American University of Beirut, and M. Hassan Murad of the Mayo Clinic. The discussion was led by planning committee member Janet A. Tooze of Wake Forest University. The discussion centered around the presentation topics and addressed questions that were asked by audience members.

Avoiding Data Errors

On the topic of ways to prevent data errors during the phases of data extraction and analysis, Akl asked Boyland about how to address complex effect modifiers. He gave the example of a WHO study on fruit and vegetable subsidies that included co-interventions such as nutrition education, which could be viewed as effect modifiers. Akl wanted to know how to best account for these effect modifiers to better understand the data. Boyland replied by urging caution during the data extraction process and suggested directly contacting study authors to better understand whether the study included control groups that were not mentioned in the final publication. Jones added that this specific example might best lend itself to a "network meta-analysis," which plots all the possible interventions and their combinations. Wells added that complex interventions may require multiple

---

[2] https://amstar.ca (accessed January 10, 2024).

methods. He said that while network MAs are useful, he has concerns about whether there would have been sufficient data in Akl's example for a network MA to be effective, as there may not have been enough evidence to run the required analysis. In complex cases where heterogeneity cannot be avoided, Wells said that teams should accept the heterogeneity, noting that it can lead to a better understanding of the effect modifier.

In response to an audience question about whether to use study data repositories or rely solely on the reports when extracting data from large epidemiological studies, Boyland noted the benefits of maximizing both volume and quality of data. Having more data to feed into the MA is a positive, and the current environment of data sharing has been an overall benefit to the MA process. Jones suggested caution with using data repositories noting that they are often sloppily organized, which can inject error. He also noted that referencing the author's report may be beneficial. Jones suggested that researchers should aim to better manage and present raw data.

Multiple audience members asked how to address the existence of multiple reports published from the same study data. If similar analyses are published in two papers from the same team, should both be included in the data synthesis or just one? If only one should be included, what criteria should guide this selection? Boyland replied that is not necessary to only use one of the data sets, but if the same data set has been analyzed in multiple ways, teams should consider which outcome to use in the MA. Those conducting the MA should be able to rely on their agreed-upon methods, PICO, and hierarchy of decision making in these cases, asking what data are most relevant to the research question and what are the most valid tools that have been used to generate the data. There are no set rules, Boyland said, but it is essential to create and adhere to guidelines for the MA. Akl agreed with Boyland, stating that it is important to consider what data have been produced using the highest quality and most appropriate methodologies and which data are the best fit for the population of interest. He added that using multiple publications based on the same data set could have an undue influence on policy development, as each paper may be interpreted by policy makers as independent evidence. It is important when doing MAs for the purpose of impacting policy, Akl said, to be sure that duplicate data is not used in a way that can bias results.

An audience member asked about including subgroups in an MA and whether a team might accidentally double- or triple-count the data from a single study. Jones asserted in response that including the same study carried out in multiple groups would violate independence principles and require a more technical, multilevel MA. However, Wells noted that there are ways to include subgroup data that do not double-count the same evidence, but they require careful planning and analysis, a point on which Tooze concurred. Wells gave the example of one of his research teams spending months analyzing this type of data, and issues arose when they tried to manipulate the data by study participant—an attempt to make the populations independent from each other. He said that when data independence is straightforward, separating groups and carrying out subgroup analyses can be effective. However, he warned that caution should be exercised when the subgroups become highly complex, and issues can arise when researchers attempt to manipulate data to this extent. He suggested the use of an Instrument for assessing the Credibility of Effect Modification Analyses (ICEMAN), which can be used to assess factors beyond statistical significance and provide analysis within or between studies. Beyene commented that meta-regression provides an advantage over subgroup analysis when exploring potential heterogeneity, especially when the factors being analyzed are continuous. The downside to such an analysis, he said, is the focus on the aggregate data, which have limitations that can be challenging to disentangle. He noted similar challenges in dose-response studies, stating that it is difficult to know whether the relationship is linear. Beyene acknowledged that there are many potential challenges with data analysis, and researchers should use their best judgment as to which method of analysis is best for their study.

Preventing and Evaluating Bias

The second discussion focused on preventing and evaluating bias in SRs and MAs. Murad noted that Boyland's presentation had a strong focus on RCTs, but there are many other study designs used in the field of nutrition research and additional tools for assessing risk of bias in other types of studies, including observational studies and case series. Although the early version of Cochrane's Risk of Bias tool mainly focused on analyzing the presence of bias in RCTs, he said that many other methods and tools have since become available.

Murad addressed Jones's presentation, stating that he feels "very pessimistic" about publication bias, given that it occurs frequently and its existence is difficult to determine, particularly when analyzing small, nonrandomized studies that have not been registered. Murad stated that conducting multiple analyses to identify the results of greatest significance, which can be done most easily with small, unregistered, non-randomized studies, poses a large threat to research that may not be easily overcome. Murad also responded to a question from an audience member about the best risk of bias tools for nutrition research considering the lack of RCTs used in the field and listed some tools that are used for non-randomized comparative studies. He spoke about the Newcastle-Ottawa Scale (NOS) tool,[3] the Cochrane Risk of Bias in Non-randomized Studies–of Exposures (ROBINS-E) tool, and the Cochrane Risk of Bias in Non-randomized Studies–of Interventions (ROBINS-I) tool. He said that ROBINS-E is usually more relevant for nutrition studies, but the tool is challenging to use and requires specific training. Murad added that specific tools exist for each type of study, and resources and trainings can help guide researchers to the right tools for their particular study.

Tooze asked a follow-up question about the use of I-squared analysis as a measure of heterogeneity in nutrition studies, inquiring whether a high I-squared value is always expected. Murad replied that a high number would be expected in an observational study, which makes the tool less useful in these cases. Akl and Wells agreed that, in this context, the I-squared value would be high and not very useful as a statistical measurement.

Interpreting Data Through Statistical Analysis

The third discussion centered on best practices for interpreting data though statistical analysis. The discussion touched on best practices for data analysis within MAs and pros and cons of conducting an MA.

Beyene asked the presenters why one would conduct an MA. Wells replied that the goal of an MA is to increase the power to answer a research question by combining studies. However, challenges with MAs include inconsistencies in data, excessive heterogeneity, and the shortcoming of certain statistical tools. He noted that in addition to combining studies and potentially gaining a better understanding of a treatment effect, MAs provide a good opportunity to explore differences between studies. In this way, Wells said, MAs are tools for both synthesizing and analyzing evidence.

Wells spoke further about addressing heterogeneity, saying that the forest plot can be a helpful visual in identifying likely heterogeneity. He said that addressing heterogeneity through statistical tools can be challenging due to the lack of strength of many of the tools or their lack of accuracy. For example, the Q-test was used for this purpose for years, but it does not test the correct hypothesis because the null hypothesis is not set up to be rejected. Instead, the goal is to not reject it to claim homogeneity. Furthermore, he noted that the Q-test does not have enough power to be a useful analysis with a small sample of studies. In these cases, he suggested that the use of the I-squared test may be more useful but noted the limitations with that method as well, which were previously mentioned by Tooze.

Furthering the discussion about heterogeneity and subgroup analyses, Tooze asked the panelists for input on the categories, such as intervention

---

[3] https://www.ohri.ca/programs/clinical_epidemiology/oxford.asp (accessed January 10, 2024).

or participant characteristics, that should be considered to reduce heterogeneity when developing the protocol. Wells replied that groups should begin with the PICO and closely examine the differences between populations with particular attention to the differences that exist across important characteristics. As nutrition interventions are often complex, Wells noted that it may be helpful to group interventions into categories to analyze them. He suggested that study duration can be a useful subgroup. Wells also noted that it can be difficult to understand the exposure in nutrition research or whether a specific intervention is causing the effect, a comment on which Murad concurred. Murad stated that in nutrition research, it is important to know exactly how much of a nutrient is leading to the change or the outcome, and he suggested using the GRADE guidance in rating certainty of evidence when interpreting dose-response studies (Murad et al., 2023). He noted that dose-response MAs are especially useful and relevant in nutrition research.

Wells detailed the statistical concept of "tau," defining it is as a "super structure" that forms within a set of data, and the study results spread out around that structure rather than around a single point. He noted that most statistical analyses of complex data sets depend on estimating tau, and for this reason, tau has become a statistical "Achilles heel." Without an accurately estimated tau, most of the complex statistical analyses will be inaccurate. Wells concluded that, in general, teams should analyze the visuals and statistical tests that are available to them and come to the best possible judgment of how to approach heterogeneity within the MA.

Murad addressed a question from an audience member about what constitutes a wide confidence interval in the context of GRADE, explaining that the modern approach is to define the effect size that is considered important. For example, if the outcome is depression, the tool used should be based on the magnitude of change that is considered by the patient to be relevant or important. Relative importance can also be driven by clinical relevance, stakeholder feedback, or statistical significance. Confidence intervals, he said, should be considered through a similarly relative context. If it crosses a predetermined, agreed-upon threshold, the confidence interval is wide. Akl added that when interpreting findings, it is important to consider clinical significance and to define a priori what is being considered as clinically significant. In the example given by Wells of the study of LSSS impacting cardiovascular health, the team defined a priori that they considered a change of 10 mmHg in a patient's blood pressure to be clinically significant. Although a change of 5 mmHg may be statistically significant, it would not meet their threshold for clinical significance. Wells agreed, adding that one should determine the minimally important difference, the effect estimate, and then the confidence interval. He suggested that the confidence interval could be positioned with respect to the clinically important difference.

Tooze relayed a question from an audience member, asking how many confounders can be included in a meta-regression and whether the answer depends on the number of studies included. Wells said that it does depend on the sample size or the number of studies included. He highlighted the ecological fallacy in which an effect may appear to exist from one study to the next, but within a single study, the effect disappears. This risk is one reason that Wells said he typically uses subgroup analyses. Most MAs are done with a smaller number of studies, and meta-regressions become an imprecise tool for analyzing a combined effect when using a small number of studies.

4

Interpretation and Application of Systematic Reviews and Meta-Analysis to Evaluate the Totality of Evidence

This chapter describes the presentations and discussions that took place during the third workshop, titled Use of Meta-Analyses in Nutrition Research and Policy: Interpretation and Application of Systematic Reviews and Meta-Analysis to Evaluate the Totality of Evidence, which took place on October 3, 2023. The overall objectives of the third workshop were to

- Recognize the impact of risk of bias and publication bias on the interpretation of study results;
- Describe the impact of data errors on the conclusions of systematic reviews (SRs) and meta-analyses (MAs);
- Describe the process of evaluating the strength of the totality of evidence; and
- Describe the different applications of SRs and MAs to research and policy development and the unique considerations for each application of evidence.

The workshop featured two main speakers, Karima Benkhedda of Health Canada and Barbara O. Schneeman of the University of California, Davis. The final workshop was moderated by planning committee member Chizuru Nishida of the World Health Organization (WHO), retired, and included a panel discussion featuring the presenters and additional discussants, Elie A. Akl of the American University in Beirut and Vasanti Malik of the University of Toronto. This final workshop in the series concluded with closing remarks from planning committee chair Katherine L. Tucker of the University of Massachusetts Lowell. Workshop speakers addressed the following questions, which were posed by the workshop sponsor in advance of the workshop:

- How to consider statistical heterogeneity when evaluating diet and disease relationships? Are higher levels of unexplained statistical heterogeneity acceptable for the field of nutrition? What are the best practices for addressing publication bias?
- How to consider risk of bias when evaluating diet and disease relationships?
- How can MA be used to evaluate the strength of the totality of evidence when there is evidence from different types of nutrition study designs?
- How can MA be used to evaluate the strength of evidence when different outcomes are reported in different studies?

FROM SCIENCE TO POLICY: EVALUATING NUTRITION EVIDENCE FOR INFORMED DECISION MAKING

Benkhedda's presentation focused on evaluating nutrition evidence for informed decision making. Her presentation covered the use of SRs and MAs for the substantiation of health claims and policy and guideline development by Health Canada as case studies to illustrate the process. Benkhedda also addressed publication bias, heterogeneity, and risk of bias evaluation and their relevance for evaluating the totality of the evidence to inform policy and guideline development. Benkhedda disclosed that she is part of the NuQuest working group that develops risk of bias assessment tools for nutrition research, and her presentation was developed using both published research and unpublished data.

Benkhedda defined a "health claim" as any presentation in labeling or advertising that states, suggests, or otherwise implies that a relationship exists between the consumption of a food or ingredient in the food and a person's health. She noted that such claims can be expressed in images or symbols and are not limited to words. Exploring Health Canada's approach to evaluating evidence to support health claims, Benkhedda spoke about two major guidance documents that are available to inform industry about how to use the literature to inform their health claims: Health Canada's Guidance Document for Preparing a Submission for Food Health Claims[1] and Health Canada's Guidance Document for Preparing a Submission for Food Health Claims

---

[1] https://www.canada.ca/en/health-canada/services/food-nutrition/legislation-guidelines/guidance-documents/guidance-document-preparing-submission-food-health-claims-2009-1.html (accessed January 10, 2024).

Using an Existing Systematic Review.[2] Benkhedda said that while SRs are required to substantiate health claims, MAs are not. However, MAs can be useful for informing the review and evaluation of evidence.

Benkhedda detailed the systematic approach required for health claim substantiation,[3] as shown in Figure 4-1. The process begins with a research question that is the basis of the claim, then follows a specific set of steps that culminates with a conclusion about the claim, development of the claim wording, and determination of the conditions under which the claim can be used.

Benkhedda explored the types of study designs that are used for the substantiation of health claims by Health Canada. She said that SRs, MAs, and randomized controlled trials (RCTs) are considered the highest level of evidence for health claims because they establish causality and provide information on intake-response relationships. She said that prospective observational studies (i.e., cohort studies and nested case-control studies) could also be included but would be considered a lower quality of evidence because they only show association, have more confounders, and cannot establish causality. She explained that prospective studies are more prone to bias, both through self-reporting and selection bias. On the topic of bias, Benkhedda added that publication bias may impact a review. Although this concern is not unique to MAs, she noted that it can be a major challenge due to the tendency to report on studies that show a significant effect. More bias can be introduced through search methods, such as language constraints or ignoring "gray" literature, which was previously described by Andrew Jones in Chapter 3. Benkhedda cautioned that having relevant studies missing from a review could adversely impact the intended decision making.

Benkhedda detailed a real-world example of an MA that was performed to examine the impact of dietary changes on low-density lipoprotein cholesterol. The MA included RCTs but contained high levels of statistical heterogeneity. In the forest plot, the studies were organized from largest to smallest effect to examine the relationship between sample size and effect size and the possibility of missing studies with small effect size or no effect, which could impact the results of the MA. To assess the absence of such studies, Benkhedda referenced the use of funnel plots, which were described by Jones in Chapter 3. Benkhedda noted that this method is imperfect and may perform poorly in settings with high heterogeneity because asymmetry in the funnel plot, which represents missing studies, can also occur because

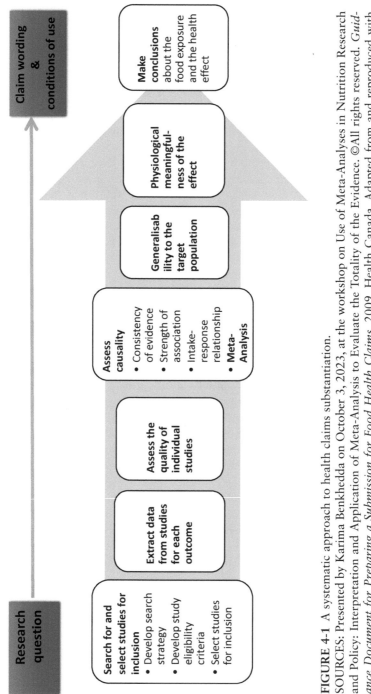

FIGURE 4-1 A systematic approach to health claims substantiation.

SOURCES: Presented by Karima Benkhedda on October 3, 2023, at the workshop on Use of Meta-Analyses in Nutrition Research and Policy: Interpretation and Application of Meta-Analysis to Evaluate the Totality of the Evidence. ©All rights reserved. *Guidance Document for Preparing a Submission for Food Health Claims*, 2009. Health Canada. Adapted from and reproduced with the permission of Health Canada, 2023. Available at the following address: https://www.canada.ca/en/health-canada/services/food-nutrition/legislation-guidelines/guidance-documents/guidance-document-preparing-submission-food-health-claims-2009-1.html (accessed January 10, 2024).

of the high heterogeneity. Benkhedda said that it was important to use additional methods of analysis to assess the quality of evidence, especially since the review would be used to inform decision making in a policy setting. She said that the team in this example also used subgroup analyses to explore the heterogeneity present in their selected studies, examining the study duration, participant demographics, and other relevant subgroups. They also tried removing studies with the strongest effects to assess the impact of their absence on the overall results of the MA. The bottom line, Benkhedda said, is that interpreting publication bias involves a combination of visual inspection of funnel plots, statistical tests, sensitivity analysis, and expert judgment.

Benkhedda addressed a question of how to consider statistical heterogeneity when evaluating diet and disease relationships, inquiring whether higher levels of unexplained statistical heterogeneity are acceptable in the nutrition field. She stated that in situations where heterogeneity cannot be explained, a decision should be made about whether to pool the data. She said that some experts warn against pooling in high heterogeneity settings due to reduced confidence in effect estimates. Benkhedda acknowledged the validity of this concern in the nutrition field, even though high heterogeneity is often expected. She added that publication bias should also be considered, suggesting that research teams consult with both research methods and subject-matter experts. She said that it is important to evaluate each study individually rather than make a general statement about allowing for high levels of heterogeneity. Poorly done studies will reduce the overall quality of evidence and introduce bias, which will negatively impact the summary effect of the MA. Benkhedda shared Figure 4-2, which details the various domains of bias that may exist in nutrition studies (Kelly et al., 2022)

As Benkhedda discussed, most risk of bias tools are not specifically designed to address the key ways in which bias can enter nutrition studies, but some tools have been adapted to address these issues. To illustrate this, she displayed the two quality appraisal tools used by Health Canada[4] shown in Figure 4-3. As Benkhedda highlighted, the quality appraisal tool for prospective observational studies, shown in Figure 4-3, includes questions such as whether the exposure was assessed more than once and whether the methodology used to measure the exposure was reported. She noted that confounders are also an area of concern in observational studies, and a question in the quality appraisal tool asks whether confounders were corrected for the study design or analysis process.

---

[4] https://www.canada.ca/en/health-canada/services/food-nutrition/legislation-guidelines/guidance-documents/guidance-document-preparing-submission-food-health-claims-2009-1.html (accessed January 10, 2024).

Performance bias	Systematic differences between groups in the care provided or exposure to factors other than the interventions/exposure of interest.
Attrition bias	Systematic differences between groups in withdrawals from the study.
Detection bias	Systematic differences between groups in how exposure/status and outcomes are determined.
Selection bias	Systematic differences between groups on baseline characteristics.
Dietary exposure assessment bias	Error associated with the use of methodologies for assessing dietary intakes. A subcategory for self-reporting methodologies is **recall bias**, which refers to systematic error due to differences in completeness or accuracy of recall. Self-reported dietary intakes are at risk of this bias.
Misclassification bias	Systematic error due to inaccurate measurements or classifications of participants' exposure or outcome; error may be related to the risk of outcome. If the error is unrelated to the risk of outcome, the effect is usually biased to the null.

FIGURE 4-2 Potential types of bias in nutrition studies.
SOURCES: Presented by Karima Benkhedda on October 3, 2023, at the workshop on Use of Meta-Analyses in Nutrition Research and Policy: Interpretation and Application of Meta-Analysis to Evaluate the Totality of the Evidence (Kelly et al., 2022). Reproduced with permission.

Quality appraisal tool for intervention studies			
Assign a score of 1 for each "Yes", and a score of 0 for each "No/NR".			
Reference (Author, year):			
Item	Question	Score	
		Yes	No/NR
1. Inclusion/ Exclusion Criteria	Were the inclusion and/or exclusion criteria for study participation reported (*e.g.*, age greater than 50 years, no history of heart disease)?		
2. Group Allocation[1]	Was the study described as randomized?		
	Was the randomization method reported?		
	Was the randomization method appropriate?[2]		
	Was allocation concealed?[3]		
3. Blinding	Were the study subjects blinded to the intervention received?		
	Were the research personnel blinded to the intervention received by the subjects?		
4. Attrition	Was attrition numerically reported?		
	Were the reasons for withdrawals and dropouts provided?[4]		
5. Exposure/ Intervention	Was the type of food described (e.g., composition, matrix)?		
	Was the amount of food described (i.e., dose)?		
6. Health Effect	Was the methodology used to measure the health effect reported?		
7. Statistical Analysis	Was a between-group statistical analysis of the health effect conducted (*i.e.*, control vs. intervention)?		
	Was an intention-to-treat analysis conducted?[5]		
8. Potential Confounders	Were potential confounders of the food/health relationship considered?[6]		
TOTAL SCORE (maximum of 15):			
Higher quality (Score ≥ 8)		☐	
Lower quality (Score ≤ 7)		☐	

FIGURE 4-3 Quality appraisal tool for intervention studies and quality appraisal tool for prospective observational studies used by Health Canada.
SOURCES: Presented by Karima Benkhedda on October 3, 2023, at the workshop on Use of Meta-Analyses in Nutrition Research and Policy: Interpretation and Application of Meta-Analysis to Evaluate the Totality of the Evidence. ©All rights reserved. *Guidance Document for Preparing a Submission for Food Health Claims*, 2009. Health Canada. Reproduced with the permission of Health Canada, 2023. Available at the following address: https://www.canada.ca/en/health-canada/services/food-nutrition/legislation-guidelines/guidance-documents/guidance-document-preparing-submission-food-health-claims-2009-1.html (accessed January 10, 2024).

continued

Quality appraisal tool for prospective observational studies			
Assign a score of 1 for each "Yes", and a score of 0 for each "No/NR".			
Reference (Author, year):			
Item	Question	Score	
		Yes	No/N R
1. Inclusion/ Exclusion Criteria	Were the inclusion and/or exclusion criteria for study participation reported (e.g., age greater than 50 years, no history of heart disease)?		
2. Attrition	Was attrition numerically reported?		
	Were the reasons for withdrawals and dropouts provided?[1]		
3. Exposure	Was the methodology used to measure the exposure reported?		
	Was the exposure assessed more than once?		
4. Health Outcome	Was the methodology used to measure the health outcome reported?		
	Was the health outcome verified (e.g., through assessment of medical records, confirmation by a health professional)?		
5. Blinding	Were the outcome assessors blinded to the exposure status?		
6. Baseline Comparability of groups	Were the subjects in the different exposure levels compared at baseline?		
7. Statistical Analysis	Was the statistical significance of the trend reported?		
8. Potential Confounders	Were key confounders related to subjects' demographics accounted for in the statistical analysis?[2,3]		
	Were key confounders related to other risk factors of the health outcome accounted for in the statistical analysis?[2,4]		
TOTAL SCORE (maximum of 12):			
Higher quality (Score ≥ 7)		☐	
Lower quality (Score ≤ 6)		☐	

FIGURE 4-3 Continued

Benkhedda described an additional example from Health Canada in which the evidence for a health claim on whole grains and coronary heart disease (CHD) was evaluated. The objective of the study was to determine whether the given evidence supported a health claim about whole grain foods and a reduced risk of CHD in the general population. The evaluation team used the Population, Intervention, Comparator, Outcome (PICO) framework to set up their SR, as shown in Box 4-1. The PICO framework was discussed in more detail by Celeste Naude in Chapter 3.

A systematic review of 26 RCTs and 6 cohort studies was conducted, and an MA of RCTs was performed for LDL and total cholesterol outcomes (Health Canada, 2012). Evidence from the RCTs showed a statistically significant effect, but when analyzing only the high-quality evidence, or the evidence on grains other than those high in beta-glucan fiber, this effect

---

BOX 4-1
PICO for Health Canada's Systematic Review on
Whole Grain Intake and Coronary Heart Disease

Population: Adults, excluding people with diabetes or coronary artery disease
Intervention: Whole grain foods or diets high in whole grain foods
Comparator: Foods or diets low in whole grains
Outcomes: Primary- CHD mortality and incidence. Secondary- change in CHD risk biomarkers such as blood pressure, cholesterol, and low-density lipoprotein

SOURCE: Presented by Karima Benkhedda on October 3, 2023, at the workshop on Use of Meta-Analyses in Nutrition Research and Policy: Interpretation and Application of Meta-Analysis to Evaluate the Totality of the Evidence.

---

was lost. The data from cohort studies was too heterogeneous to be pooled, and most of the studies were deemed to be too low quality with a high risk of bias due to lack of adjustment for confounders and lack of control for potential confounders. In the end, the evidence was not sufficient to support a health claim about whole grains and CHD risk reduction.

Benkhedda addressed the question of how to consider risk of bias when evaluating diet and disease relationships. She stated the importance of considering the overall quality of evidence and referenced the previous example of the MA on whole grain intake and CHD in which the evidence was not considered high enough quality to substantiate a claim. Referring to Figure 4-1, which depicts Health Canada's approach to health claims substantiation, Benkhedda spoke about ways to assess causality, including considering the overall consistency of the evidence, the strength of association, and the intake-response (or dose-response) relationships. She explained that MAs can help to determine health claim validity by assessing these factors and the overall quality of evidence across studies. MAs can answer questions such as whether consistency was high across the higher quality studies and if appropriate tests were used to quantify heterogeneity. Benkhedda suggested analyzing the proportion of studies that showed statistically significant effects and explore their quality and what factors might have impacted the statistical significance of the nonsignificant studies. Benkhedda said that when considering dose-response relationships, the minimum effective amount shown to produce a response should be identified, and in observational studies, statistically significant differences found between the highest intake groups and lowest intake groups should be examined.

Benkhedda spoke about the importance of assessing the generalizability and relevance of study data to the general population when looking to inform guideline and policy development. One question to consider is whether the population studied is representative of the general population. Benkhedda emphasized the importance of establishing the applicability of the MA results to the target population, and for health claims, the target population is the general population of the country. Doing subgroup analyses within the MA can help to establish the robustness of the effect for important subgroups of interest with a focus on the physiological meaningfulness of a food's effect. Questions to consider include whether the observed effects have clinical relevance and whether the effect disappears within a few weeks or months or is durable long-term. Benkhedda highlighted the importance of quantifying the impact of the food exposure on human health.

Addressing a question of how MAs can be used to evaluate the strength of the totality of evidence when the evidence comes from different types of nutrition study designs, Benkhedda reiterated the benefits of a broad, holistic assessment of evidence. Consider the comprehensiveness, relevant outcomes, consistency and strength of association, quality, meaningfulness of the effect size, and the generalizability of the data, she suggested.

Benkhedda also addressed the question of how MAs can be used to evaluate the strength of the evidence when different outcomes are reported in different studies. To this, Benkhedda said that claim wording should reflect the specific evidence. For example, the claim should reflect whether the evidence showed prevention of disease, change in disease outcome, or change in disease risk biomarkers. She illustrated this point with another real-world example. Health Canada examined the evidence to support a health claim for fruit and vegetable consumption to reduce the risk of heart disease and examined evidence to support a health claim of whole grains consumption to reduce CHD risk. They found sufficient evidence to support the health claims for fruits and vegetables but did not find sufficient evidence to support the health claims for whole grains. The lack of sufficient evidence was due to the fact that a sensitivity analysis revealed the evidence for the whole grains health claim was in limited trials on grains high in beta-glucan and in studies judged to be of poor quality, which were credited with producing most of the effect.

Benkhedda concluded her presentation with a general overview of the considerations for use of MA in policy development. She suggested using the best evidence available, including SRs, MAs, and other relevant individual studies. Considerations should be given to the relevance of a study to the specific policy question, the overall quality of evidence, the level of certainty, and the applicability of the evidence to the general population in a national context. The advantage of MAs and SRs, she noted, is that they examine a large sample of studies under similar conditions and can draw conclusions that are relevant to policy development. However, Benkhedda noted that the included research should be relevant to the policy question, and she suggested that it may be helpful to conduct SRs in collaboration with policy makers.

NUTRITION AND POLICY: EVALUATING THE EVIDENCE

Barbara O. Schneeman's presentation focused on examples of the application of MAs and SRs in nutrition policy. She featured examples across three bodies that use nutrition research to develop guidelines and policies: the U.S. Food and Drug Administration (FDA), the U.S. Dietary Guidelines Advisory Committee (DGAC), and the WHO Nutrition Guidance Expert Advisory Group Subcommittee (NUGAG). Specifically, she addressed FDA's use of SR evidence in acceptance, denial, or qualification of health claims; DGAC's use of SR evidence to produce DGAC reports to advise the relevant federal agencies on updates to the *Dietary Guidelines for Americans* (DGA); and WHO's use of SRs and MAs in the development of nutrition guidelines. Schneeman disclosed that she holds, or has held, affiliations with numerous stakeholder organizations, including DGAC, WHO NUGAG, National Academies of Sciences, Engineering, and Medicine's Food and Nutrition Board, and the International Union of Food Science and Technology Task Force on Food Classification. She also noted her position as an advisory board member, and/or member of the board of trustees for organizations including the International Food Information Council, McCormick Science Institute, and the Coalition for Grain Fiber Science Advisory Committee.

Schneeman provided WHO's definitions of SR and MA. As she quoted, "an SR is a review of a clearly formulated question that uses systematic and explicit methods to identify, select, and critically appraise relevant research and to extract and analyze data from the studies that are included in a review" (WHO, 2014). An SR is different from an MA, which refers to the quantitative synthesis, or pooling, of outcome data across comparable studies to achieve a pooled estimate of effect (WHO, 2014). Schneeman explained that if data from an SR meets certain requirements, such as high homogeneity across study design, population, and intervention, then the data can be combined into an MA. An MA can also be distinguished from an SR in that an MA is a statistical method that provides a summary estimate of effect across a body of evidence.

Schneeman described the process of undertaking an SR by each of the three authoritative bodies. At FDA, this process is initiated in response to a petition or when the agency considers updating existing claims. A scoping review is useful to determine whether there are any major and relevant omissions in the literature submitted with a petition. The DGAC uses SRs to review the evidence on topics for inclusion in the next iteration of the DGA, and the U.S. Department of Agriculture's (USDA's) Nutrition Evidence Systematic Review (NESR) team[5] has proposed using scoping reviews to identify potential topics for the DGA. At WHO, an SR is used to identify the availability of relevant evidence for guideline development and to facilitate protocol development.

Schneeman detailed the process of structuring an SR and an MA. She noted that her description would not be comprehensive but instead illustrative for the topic of interest. She stated that research teams should identify the population of interest, including characteristics such as age, sex, and health status, and the intervention or exposure, aiming for specificity to allow for identification of studies that are relevant to the policy question. She noted that for health claims, FDA would be particularly interested in the impact of a substance compared to the lack of that substance. Likewise, for dietary guidelines the nature of the comparison is important. For example, when considering the impact of saturated fat intake on health outcomes, reviewers must consider the comparison group, such as low fat, other types of fat, or carbohydrates. It is a challenge, Schneeman noted, to be clear about the exact nature of the intervention, the control, and the comparison.

Schneeman explained the importance of identifying the outcomes of interest for the review and how to decide what evidence to include and exclude from the review. As mentioned by Naude and Hooper in Chapter 2, having protocols in place can be beneficial for ensuring that all decision-making criteria are consistently applied. Specific, meaningful outcomes are important when evaluating evidence for health claims, Schneeman said. She emphasized that it is critical to consider the intended use of evidence and which studies are and are not relevant to the research question. For example, when developing dietary guidelines for the national population, a study that showed the clinical impact of a dietary intervention used to treat a disease may be relevant to evaluate clinical treatments but not relevant for developing policies to reduce risk for a disease.

Schneeman noted that it is important for policy makers to understand the overall quality of evidence and whether it results in significant scientific agreement. To this end, Schneeman described how an MA can provide insight into the inconsistencies in the available evidence. As described by Wells in Chapter 3, Schneeman noted that MAs can be used to examine the differences between studies. She restated the usefulness of subgroup analyses, previously explained by Jones and Wells in Chapter 3, when subgroups are relevant to the specific guidelines being developed. She noted that DGAC and the USDA NESR team provide an analytical framework for

---

[5] For information on NESR, see https://nesr.usda.gov/ (accessed January 10, 2024).

understanding the key factors that may impact the relationships in nutrition studies, such as confounders, covariates, and moderators.

Schneeman described the processes of structuring an SR at the three entities of focus. At FDA, when an SR is developed in response to a health claim petition or as evidence for food labeling, the petition will be used to create the PICO elements, and the inclusion and exclusion criteria are specified in the FDA guidance document.[6] For DGAC, NESR methodology specifies the inclusion and exclusion criteria that will be used in the SR, which must be relevant to the DGA and may be modified as needed by DGAC to address specific questions. The SR is conducted by methodological experts. Figure 4-4 displays the steps used by DGAC to implement NESR's process[7] for planning and executing an SR. When an SR is performed for WHO NUGAG, the subcommittee determines the PICO elements, identifies the outcomes that are critical for decision making, and specifies the inclusion and exclusion criteria using an approach that is consistent with the WHO Guideline Development handbook (WHO, 2014). Overall, Schneeman reinforced the importance of bringing methodology and subject-matter experts into every level of the process.

Schneeman discussed the methods for determining the strength of the evidence and how these processes differ across the three governing bodies. At FDA, the focus is on whether the evidence is consistent with significant scientific agreement. DGAC assigns each SR a grade with criteria for risk of bias, consistency, precision, directness, and generalizability. WHO uses the Grading of Recommendations Assessment, Development and Evaluation (GRADE) methodology for rating evidence, which considers study design and allows for researchers to evaluate and grade the quality of their evidence on a rating scale from very high-quality evidence to very low-quality evidence. This approach, Schneeman said, may help to improve objectivity when assessing the strength of the evidence.

After grading and analyzing the evidence, Schneeman explained, the next phase is the decision-making process, a step that she described as critical but often overlooked. She explained that this phase of the process is where the three groups most differ in their approach. At FDA, the criteria and conditions related to the food products that might bear a claim must be considered as well as the legal and economic factors on the use of claims in labeling. DGAC considers not only the evidence from SRs for its conclusions but also data analysis from National Health and Nutrition Examination Survey to understand current intakes as well as food pattern modeling to structure healthful dietary patterns. Schneeman explained that

---

[6] For the FDA guidance document, see https://www.fda.gov/food/food-labeling-nutrition/qualified-health-claims (accessed January 10, 2024).

[7] https://nesr.usda.gov/ (accessed January 10, 2024).

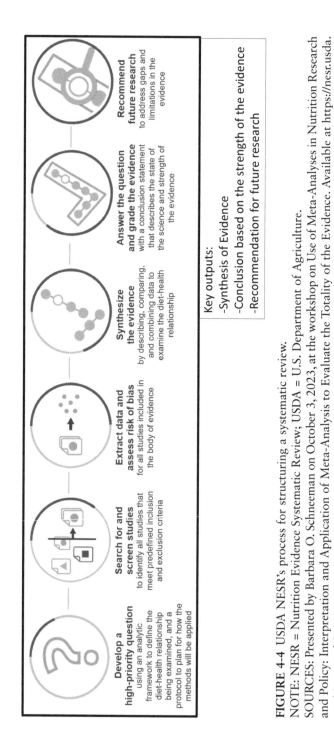

FIGURE 4-4 USDA NESR's process for structuring a systematic review.

NOTE: NESR = Nutrition Evidence Systematic Review; USDA = U.S. Department of Agriculture.

SOURCES: Presented by Barbara O. Schneeman on October 3, 2023, at the workshop on Use of Meta-Analyses in Nutrition Research and Policy: Interpretation and Application of Meta-Analysis to Evaluate the Totality of the Evidence. Available at https://nesr.usda. gov/ (accessed January 10, 2024).

DGAC integrates the evidence from these three approaches to develop its conclusions. For example, the evidence from SRs to support the DGA recommendation on added sugars was graded as limited and insufficient. However, examining food pattern modeling allowed DGAC to estimate the extent to which added sugars could be consumed while maintaining a healthful dietary pattern. This additional information allowed DGAC to conclude that typical dietary intakes could be improved by recommending a limit to added sugars intake. DGAC was able to come to this conclusion by integrating the full body of evidence. At WHO, SRs and MAs are integrated into decision making using a series of contextual factors to determine the strength of the recommendations. For example, WHO considers the balance of benefits and harms, resource implications, confidence in effect estimates, equity and human rights, accessibility, and feasibility.

Schneeman shared some observations from her experiences using MA in the decision-making process. She stated that a well-designed SR is essential for a proper MA. She recommended having experts in methodology involved in designing the SR and performing the MA. She also recommended conducting a scoping review prior to an SR to set the parameters for the SR and focus on the information that is critical to the decision making. Schneeman said that SRs should be designed to fit the specific purpose of the policy or guidance, and MAs should allow for a deeper examination of the evidence to better understand the strength of the evidence. Again, she noted that subgroup analyses can assist with addressing and understanding high levels of heterogeneity. She also noted that MAs can provide a more objective assessment of the strength of the evidence, making them a useful tool. However, Schneeman said, when MAs are not possible, other tools can be used such as harvest plots. Harvest plots are often used when creating nutrition policy and guidelines in conditions where MAs are not an appropriate tool.

Schneeman provided a brief overview of the opportunities and challenges for using MAs to develop guidance across the three governing bodies profiled. She suggested that, at FDA, a graphic display (e.g., a forest plot) might better illustrate the balance of evidence and be a useful tool to clarify inconsistencies in the current evidence. For DGAC, MAs could provide more transparency when rating the strength of the evidence. She also suggested that nonqualitative summary tools could facilitate recommendations related to the food environment and policy and that subgroup analysis could better help the committee understand which subgroups would benefit most from specific changes to the DGA. Schneeman noted that MAs are used for guideline development at WHO, which allows for experts in methodology to assess the strength of the evidence and for expert guidance committees to use the MAs in the development of the recommendation.

She pointed out that MAs could also be used to determine when evidence is insufficient to produce a recommendation.

PANEL DISCUSSION

Nishida led a panel discussion featuring Benkhedda and Schneeman, who were joined by Malik and Akl.

Tools to Assess the Quality of Nutrition Research to Inform Policy

A question posed by planning committee member Russell Jude de Souza, and echoed by other audience members, asked whether the field of nutrition is so unique that it requires its own set of statistical and analytical tools. Nishida further inquired whether there are formal criteria for use of existing tools that would make them more effective in nutrition research for policy development. Akl replied, disclosing that his role as part of the GRADE working group has informed his perspective, and said that while many fields may consider theirs to be unique, his opinion is that the principles should be the same across fields. Whether a research team uses GRADE or Nutri-Grade to assess their evidence, the result should be the same. The general principles across fields are that certainty in effect estimates is affected by risk of bias, inconsistency of results, imprecision, indirect evidence, and publication bias. However, Akl said, in certain fields small effect sizes may be more meaningful. For example, in public health, a small effect size across a large population could lead to a meaningful public health impact. What is judged as a small effect size in one field might be considered significant in another field.

Akl described additional factors that he thinks are particularly relevant to the nutrition field. For example, in nutrition it is common to have outcomes with continuous measurements. Continuous scales often show heterogeneity due to the nature of the data. This factor should be considered when assessing heterogeneity in nutrition research, Akl said, and not "over-rated," which could lead to the downgrading of the certainty of evidence. He referred to Schneeman's comment about fitting the method to the purpose, further emphasizing that "the method should fit the purpose of the eventual product." He noted that FDA and DGAC use different approaches for different goals: validation of health claims and development of guidelines, respectively. Akl highlighted that the involvement of content experts in the development and use of SRs and MAs is important, a point on which Malik concurred. Akl noted that experts are important for judging effect sizes and non-health effects.

Akl also encouraged the consideration of the contextual factors that impact nutrition policy and guideline development, such as the resources that would be required to implement or enforce a policy or recommendation and the acceptance of a recommendation to stakeholders such as industry and consumers. He urged researchers to consider the real-world implications of a potential policy or guideline, suggesting that SRs that examine these contextual factors could be part of the methodologies that governing bodies use to inform their process. Akl noted that Health Canada's process of analyzing research to inform policy development, as described by Benkhedda, is an excellent example of the consistent and effective use of existing research tools.

Malik suggested that the "hierarchy of evidence" pyramid, as shown in Figure 4-5, which was presented by Benkhedda and is commonly used when evaluating quality of evidence, may not be the ideal reference point for the field of nutrition (Yetley et al., 2017). Nishida concurred with this comment. Malik suggested that, given that the field of nutrition often examines longitudinal relationships between diet and health, a restructuring of the pyramid should be considered. Currently, RCTs are the highest level of evidence and cohort studies are viewed as lower quality; Malik suggested that they could be shown side by side. When it comes to nutrition, longitudinal cohort studies are often better able to truly examine longitudinal relationships, and it is typically not feasible to use RCTs for this purpose. Blinding is also not possible in most nutrition studies.

Benkhedda agreed that sometimes well-designed and well-conducted observational studies do yield better results than poor-quality RCTs. However, she noted that in validating health claims, Health Canada requires RCTs first and then observational studies can provide additional support. If an observational study shows an effect, a follow-up RCT on the food or nutrient in question can help to clarify and determine whether a causal relationship truly exists. However, she agreed that for dietary guideline development, RCTs may not be the most important source of data, suggesting that further discussion on this topic among nutrition experts may be warranted.

Schneeman stated that the GRADE approach can be helpful because it allows for the upgrading or downgrading of certain studies relative to their efficacy in answering the research question. According to Schneeman, the nutrition field does not need new or unique tools but can use existing tools to rate evidence as accurately as possible. She also emphasized that different government bodies, and different countries, have specific legal and contextual factors to consider when developing nutrition policy. For example, in the United States, the First Amendment is a consideration in the health claim process. RCTs may still be required to verify health claims. Schneeman added that while she used to think nutrition studies were unique in their complexity and required unique tools, her thinking has evolved over her career, and she has come to understand that using well-defined tools consistently over time to facilitate improved understanding of the data can contribute to effective policy decision making as well as to transparency in the decision-making process.

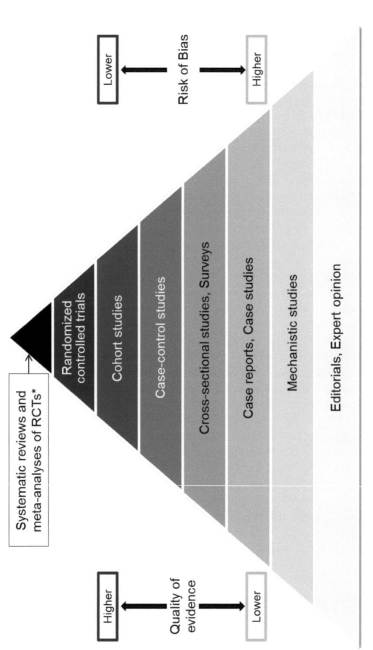

FIGURE 4-5 A hierarchy of evidence for health claims substantiation used by Health Canada.
SOURCES: Presented by Karima Benkhedda on October 3, 2023, at the workshop on Use of Meta-Analyses in Nutrition Research and Policy: Interpretation and Application of Meta-Analysis to Evaluate the Totality of the Evidence (Yetley et al., 2017).

Benkhedda and Malik added their agreement with Schneeman and Akl that the consistent use of existing tools is key to their efficacy. Benkhedda also noted that many recent publications have initiated discussions to address consistency and quality of data and appropriate data analysis tools in the field of nutrition research. For example, one common problem is the lack of appropriate risk of bias tools that work with the common study types used in nutrition research. These tools can be adapted but may not work consistently across SRs and MAs, which limits how researchers can interpret bias in nutrition studies.

Conflict of Interest and Bias

The second major topic of conversation was the potential impacts of conflict of interest, including funding sources and other vested interests, on nutrition research results and ways to mitigate this bias. Benkhedda explained Health Canada's approach for health claims validation, stating that Health Canada examines evidence through a set of objective criteria, and that while they do not exclude evidence due to funding source, they evaluate the merit of the study based on the same objective criteria used to evaluate all studies. Health Canada also considers whether the funding source may have influenced the outcome of the study. For nutrition guidelines, Benkhedda noted that the committee developing the guideline may choose to exclude studies funded by industry.

Akl added that funding by industry or an interested party, or a conflict of interest from study authors, does not necessarily negatively impact a study; but it has to predict when it would and when it would not. Therefore, these represent a "red flag" that should be attended to because evidence shows that studies funded by industry have more favorable results than those that are not. He also explained that conflicts of interest can exist beyond funding, such as intellectual conflicts of interest among members of a committee or a reviewing body. If an expert comes to a panel with a preconceived notion about a recommendation, Akl explained, they may not have an open mind about the evidence being presented. This type of conflict of interest can be very challenging to detect, as it falls outside the standard conflict of interest declaration and management policies.

Schneeman added that for health claims and petitions to FDA, most of the evidence provided will be funded by industry. However, the evidence must still meet prespecified transparent criteria, which are created to ensure that the evidence is high quality.

Malik added that she has found it useful in her experience as a researcher managing MAs to conduct a subgroup analysis by funding source. Also, the Nutri-Grade system has the option to screen data by funding source when using the tool to rank evidence in an MA.

5

Closing Remarks

Each of the three workshops concluded with closing remarks. The closing speaker for the first workshop was Mei Chung from Tufts University. The second workshop ended with remarks from Russell de Souza of McMaster University. The third workshop concluded with comments from Katherine Tucker of the University of Massachusetts, Lowell. Tucker also provided the final remarks for the entire workshop series.

Tucker thanked the U.S. Food and Drug Administration for sponsoring the workshop series and for providing the guiding questions that framed the presentations; the staff from the National Academies' Food and Nutrition Board for planning and organizing the workshop series; and the workshop panelists and discussants, who both provided detailed presentations and contributed meaningfully to the discussion portions of each workshop. On behalf of the planning committee, she thanked the audience members for attending, and for contributing questions to the panel discussions.

TAKEAWAYS FROM THE WORKSHOP SERIES

As described by Tucker in the closing remarks for the workshop series, the field of nutrition research is complex and requires unique considerations. The workshop series provided discussions on strategies for maximizing the utility of systematic reviews (SRs) and meta-analyses (MAs) to inform nutrition policy. She referenced the first workshop, quoting Hooper who stated that conducting an MA is easy, but doing one well is difficult. Tucker said that nutrition research is highly complex, and policy makers cannot easily individually assess a multiplicity of studies to inform their work. Instead, they use systematic approaches such as those explained by workshop speakers throughout the series. She spoke about how nutrition research is often used to inform policy and guidelines and thus has real-life impact. Tucker emphasized the importance of systematic, consistent approaches in nutrition research, SRs, and MAs.

Tucker briefly recapped workshop one, noting Naude's discussion of best practices for planning SRs and MAs, and Hooper's discussion of best practices for methods and tools to reduce the risk of bias. Tucker then spoke about workshop two, highlighting Jones's presentation on screening data for errors and avoiding publication bias. She also touched on Boyland's presentation, which detailed the available tools that allow for risk of bias assessments and how to interpret the results of an MA. Tucker briefly discussed the presentation from Wells, which explored the statistical tools used in MA and described how to assess and address heterogeneity.

Finally, Tucker gave an overview of the presentations in workshop three given by Benkhedda and Schneeman. She spoke about Benkhedda's description of Health Canada's approach for developing guidance using evidence and the importance of using subgroup analysis to address heterogeneity. She also reinforced the benefits of appropriate and consistent use of high-quality appraisal and analysis tools. Tucker noted Schneeman's discussion of critical frameworks, such as Population, Intervention, Control, and Outcome (PICO) and Nutrition Evidence Systematic Review (NESR) methodology, and how they are used across agencies to assess the strength of evidence for developing nutrition policies.

Tucker closed by expressing her appreciation for the discussions that took place across the workshop series.

References

Boyland, E., L. McGale, M. Maden, J. Hounsome, A. Boland, K. Angus, and A. Jones. 2022. Association of food and nonalcoholic beverage marketing with children and adolescents' eating behaviors and health: A systematic review and meta-analysis. *JAMA Pediatrics* 176(7):e221037.

Brand, A., M. E. Visser, A. Schoonees, and C. E. Naude. 2022. Replacing salt with low-sodium salt substitutes (LSSS) for cardiovascular health in adults, children and pregnant women. *Cochrane Database of Systematic Reviews* 8(8):CD015207. https://doi.org/10.1002/14651858.CD015207.

DeVito, N. J., and B. Goldacre. 2019. Catalogue of bias: Publication bias. *BMJ Evidence Based Medicine* 24(2):53-54.

Ferguson, C. J., and M. T. Brannick. 2012. Publication bias in psychological science: Prevalence, methods for identifying and controlling, and implications for the use of meta-analyses. *Psychological Methods* 17(1):120-128.

Health Canada. 2009. Guidance document for preparing a submission for food health claims. Health Canada. Bureau of Nutritional Sciences. https://www.canada.ca/en/health-canada/services/food-nutrition/legislation-guidelines/guidance-documents/guidance-document-preparing-submission-food-health-claims-2009-1.html (accessed February 25, 2024).

Health Canada. 2012. Summary of Health Canada's assessment of a health claim about whole grains and coronary heart disease. Health Canada. Bureau of Nutritional Sciences. https://www.canada.ca/en/health-canada/services/food-nutrition/food-labelling/health-claims/assessments/assessment-health-claim-about-whole-grains-coronary-heart-disease.html (accessed December 31, 2023).

Kelly, S. E., L. S. Greene-Finestone, E. A. Yetley, K. Benkhedda, S. P. J. Brooks, G. A. Wells, and A. J. MacFarlane. 2022. NUQUEST—NUtrition QUality Evaluation Strengthening Tools: Development of tools for the evaluation of risk of bias in nutrition studies. *The American Journal of Clinical Nutrition* 115(1):256-271.

Murad, M. H., J. Verbeek, L. Schwingshackl, T. Filippini, M. Vinceti, E. A. Akl, R. L. Morgan, R. A. Mustafa, D. Zeraatkar, E. Senerth, R. Street, L. Lin, Y. Falck-Ytter, G. Guyatt, H. J. Schunemann, and GRADE Working Group. 2023. GRADE guidance 38: Updated guidance for rating up certainty of evidence due to a dose-response gradient. *Journal of Clinical Epidemiology* 164:45-53.

Olkin, I., I. J. Dahabreh, and T. A. Trikalinos. 2012. GOSH—A graphical display of study heterogeneity. *Research Synthesis Methods* 3(3):214-223.

Polanin, J. R., E. E. Tanner-Smith, and E. A. Hennessy. 2016. Estimating the difference between published and unpublished effect sizes: A meta-review. *Review of Educational Research* 86(1):207-236.

Schunemann, H., J. Brozek, G. Guyatt, and A. Oxman. 2013. GRADE handbook. https://gdt.gradepro.org/app/handbook/handbook.html#h.m938505z3li7 (accessed January 10, 2024).

Tarabashkina, L., P. Quester, and R. Crouch. 2016. Food advertising, children's food choices and obesity: Interplay of cognitive defenses and product evaluation: An experimental study. *International Journal of Obesity (London)* 40(4):581-586.

Tarabashkina, L., P. Quester, O. Tarabashkina, and M. Proksch. 2018. When persuasive intent and product's healthiness make a difference for young consumers. *Young Consumers* 19(1):38-54.

Terrin, N., C. H. Schmid, and J. Lau. 2005. In an empirical evaluation of the funnel plot, researchers could not visually identify publication bias. *Journal of Clinical Epidemiology* 58(9):894-901.

WHO (World Health Organization). 2014. Handbook for guideline development. 2nd edition. Geneva: World Health Organization. https://www.who.int/publications/i/item/9789241548960 (accessed January 10, 2024).

WHO. 2023. Saturated fatty acid and trans-fatty acid intake for adults and children: WHO guideline. Geneva: World Health Organization. https://www.who.int/publications/i/item/9789240073630 (accessed January 10, 2024).

Yetley, E. A., A. J. MacFarlane, L. S. Greene-Finestone, C. Garza, J. D. Ard, S. A. Atkinson, D. M. Bier, A. L. Carriquiry, W. R. Harlan, D. Hattis, J. C. King, D. Krewski, D. L. O'Connor, R. L. Prentice, J. V. Rodricks, and G. A. Wells. 2017. Options for basing Dietary Reference Intakes (DRIs) on chronic disease endpoints: Report from a joint U.S.-/Canadian-sponsored working group. *American Journal of Clinical Nutrition* 105(1):249S-285S.

A

Workshop Agendas

USE OF META-ANALYSES IN NUTRITION RESEARCH
AND POLICY: A WORKSHOP SERIES

WORKSHOP 1
USE OF META-ANALYSES IN NUTRITION RESEARCH
AND POLICY: PLANNING OF META-ANALYSIS
Virtual workshop

September 19, 2023

12:00   Welcome
         Katherine L. Tucker, *University of Massachusetts Lowell;*
         Planning Committee Chair

12:05   Sponsor Remarks
         Sarah Gebauer, *U.S. Food and Drug Administration, Center for*
         Food Safety and Applied Nutrition
         Crystal Rivers, *U.S. Food and Drug Administration, Center for*
         Food Safety and Applied Nutrition

12:20   Presentations
         Moderator
         Amanda J. MacFarlane, *Texas A&M University; Planning Committee Member*
         Presenters
         Systematic Reviews and Meta-Analysis for Developing Nutrition Guidance: The Core Pillars of Planning and Methods to Deliver High-Quality, Useful Synthesized Evidence
         Part 1: The Planning Pillars
         Celeste Naude, *Stellenbosch University*
         Part 2: The Methods Pillars to Reduce Risk of Bias
         Lee Hooper, *University of East Anglia*

1:20   Panel Discussion
         Lee Hooper, *University of East Anglia*
         Celeste Naude, *Stellenbosch University*
         Sydne Newberry, *RAND Corporation*
         Christopher Schmid, *Brown University School of Public Health*

1:50   Closing Remarks
         Mei Chung, *Tufts University; Planning Committee Member*

WORKSHOP 2
USE OF META-ANALYSES IN NUTRITION RESEARCH AND POLICY: BEST PRACTICES OF CONDUCTING META-ANALYSIS

Virtual workshop

September 25, 2023

12:00   Welcome
         Janet A. Tooze, *Wake Forest University; Planning Committee Member*

12:10   Presentations
         Moderator
         Janet A. Tooze, *Wake Forest University; Planning Committee Member*
         Presenters
         Best Practices of Meta-Analysis in Nutrition Research: A Case Study of Food Marketing Evidence to Inform Policy Guidelines
         Emma Boyland, *University of Liverpool*

Andrew Jones, *Liverpool John Moores University*
Interpreting the Results of Meta-Analyses and Addressing
Heterogeneity
George A. Wells, *University of Ottawa*

1:10   Panel Discussion
Elie A. Akl, *American University of Beirut*
Joseph Beyene, *McMaster University*
Emma Boyland, *University of Liverpool*
Andrew Jones, *Liverpool John Moores University*
M. Hassan Murad, *Mayo Clinic*
George A. Wells, *University of Ottawa*

1:50   Closing Remarks
Russell Jude de Souza, *McMaster University*; *Planning
Committee Member*

WORKSHOP 3
USE OF META-ANALYSES IN NUTRITION RESEARCH AND
POLICY: INTERPRETATION AND APPLICATION OF META-
ANALYSIS TO EVALUATE THE TOTALITY OF EVIDENCE

Virtual workshop

October 3, 2023

12:00   Welcome
Chizuru Nishida, *World Health Organization, Retired*; *Planning
Committee Member*

12:10   Presentations
Moderator
Chizuru Nishida, *World Health Organization, Retired*; *Planning
Committee Member*
Presenters
From Science to Policy: Evaluating Nutrition Evidence for
Informed Decision Making
Karima Benkhedda, *Health Canada*
Nutrition and Policy: Evaluating the Evidence
Barbara O. Schneeman, *University of California, Davis*

1:10   Panel Discussion
          Elie A. Akl, *American University of Beirut*
          Karima Benkhedda, *Health Canada*
          Vasanti Malik, *University of Toronto*
          Barbara O. Schneeman, *University of California, Davis*

1:50   Closing Remarks
          Katherine L. Tucker, *University of Massachusetts Lowell;*
          Planning Committee Chair

B

Speaker and Moderator Biographies

Elie A. Akl, Ph.D., M.P.H., M.D., is a tenured professor of medicine at the American University of Beirut, Lebanon. He serves as the associate dean for clinical research at the Faculty of Medicine, leads the division of General Internal Medicine and Geriatrics at the American University of Beirut (AUB) Medical Center, directs the AUB GRADE Center, and codirects the Center for Systematic Reviews of Health Policy and Systems Research. He has a part-time appointment in the Department of Health Research Methods, Evidence, and Impact at McMaster University. His research expertise is in systematic reviews, practice guidelines, and conflicts of interest. He serves as a guideline methodologist for several North American professional organizations and the World Health Organization. He has published more than 500 peer-reviewed papers and has been listed as a one of the "Highly Cited Researchers" yearly since 2015.

Karima Benkhedda, Ph.D., is the head of the Nutrition Quality and Safety Section in the Bureau of Nutritional Sciences, Food Directorate at Health Canada. Since joining Health Canada in 2005, Dr. Benkhedda has worked in several areas, including nutrition research, nutrition premarket assessment of supplemented foods, novel foods, food additives, fibers, and health claim substantiation. She has been extensively involved in policy and regulatory work related to supplemented foods and health claims and developing guidance on scientific requirements for health claim substantiation. Dr. Benkhedda conducted and used systematic reviews and meta-analyses in the context of food health claim review and approval and for developing guidance, policy, and regulations. She is a core member of the NuQuest

Working Group that developed risk of bias assessment tools for nutrition studies. Dr. Benkhedda has also contributed to international nutrition policy, including the Dietary Reference Intakes Nomination Process and the Codex Alimentarius Commission for the development of international food standards. She received the 2022 Assistant Deputy Minister's Award for Excellence in Science and the 2015 Assistant Deputy Minister's Award for Transparency and Openness.

Joseph Beyene, Ph.D., is a professor of biostatistics and the inaugural John D. Cameron Endowed Chair in the Genetic Determinants of Chronic Diseases, Department of Health Research Methods, Evidence, and Impact, McMaster University, Canada. He obtained his Ph.D. in biostatistics from the University of Toronto. Dr. Beyene's research interests focus on methodology development for evidence synthesis with application to public health sciences and clinical medicine; integrative statistical methods for high-dimensional data with emphasis on "multi-omics" studies; and general statistical methods for clinical trials and observational study designs. His scientific and clinical application areas span a wide range of disciplines, including maternal-child health, nutrition, and rheumatology. He has authored or coauthored more than 350 peer-reviewed scientific articles and book chapters across the areas of his training and research interest. In addition to maintaining an active methodological research program, Dr. Beyene is also involved in mentorship and supervision at various levels.

Emma Boyland, Ph.D., is a professor of food marketing and child health based in the Department of Psychology at the University of Liverpool, where she is research lead for the department and leads the Appetite and Obesity Research group. As an experimental psychologist, her work principally focuses on the food environment, characterizing the foods and beverages available, how they are marketed, and how these factors impact eating behaviors (particularly in children). She has extensive experience of knowledge translation and exchange, supporting use of evidence to inform policy progress in the United Kingdom and internationally. Dr. Boyland is an established global leader in her research field and has authored more than 120 peer-reviewed journal articles to date, as well as multiple World Health Organization reports and book chapters. She has received more than £4 million in research funding to her institution from funders, including the National Institute for Health and Care Research, the Medical Research Council, the Economic and Social Research Council, and the Wellcome Trust.

Mei Chung, Ph.D., M.P.H., is an associate professor at the Friedman School of Nutrition Science and Policy of Tufts University. Before her transition to the university, Dr. Chung was an assistant director of the Agency for Healthcare Research and Quality–designated Evidence-based Practice Center at Tufts Medical Center. She has more than a decade of experience in conducting rigorous evidence synthesis across wide ranges of health questions. She also has expertise in developing new methods and adapting existing methods of evidence synthesis to enable or facilitate the translation of evidence to policy. Dr. Chung holds a Ph.D. in nutritional epidemiology from Tufts University and an M.P.H. from Boston University.

Russell Jude de Souza, Sc.D., R.D., is a registered dietitian and associate professor in the Department of Health Research Methods, Evidence, and Impact at McMaster University. His nutritional epidemiology research program addresses the role of diet in chronic disease prevention throughout the lifespan, methodological issues related to study design, evidence synthesis and quality of evidence, and developing and applying state-of-the-art and established approaches to assessing food/diet-health associations. His methodological expertise has been recognized by local, national, and international health organizations, including service as an external resource person to the World Health Organization's Nutrition Guidelines Advisory Committee, appointment to the Nutrition Science Advisory Committee (Health Canada), a co-opted member of the Scientific Advisory Committee on Nutrition Subgroup on the Framework for the Evaluation of Evidence (Public Health England), and chairs the methodology group of the Precision Medicine in Diabetes Initiative (American Diabetes Association). He has more than 180 lifetime publications, including several in high-impact general medical journals, such as *BMJ, JAMA, JAMA Internal Medicine, Circulation*, and *Annals of Internal Medicine*; and high-impact nutrition journals, such as *Advances in Nutrition, American Journal of Clinical Nutrition, Current Developments in Nutrition*, and *Proceedings of the Nutrition Society*. He has a cumulative h-index of 59 through 2023. He is a member of the Canadian Nutrition Society, American Society for Nutrition, the College of Dietitians of Ontario, and Dietitians of Canada. He holds a B.A. from Queen's University (1996), bachelor of applied science in foods and nutrition from Toronto Metropolitan University (1999), an M.S. in nutritional sciences from the University of Toronto (2005), and an Sc.D. from the Harvard T.H. Chan School of Public Health (2011). He completed his graduate dietetic internship at St. Michael's Hospital, Toronto, Ontario (2000).

Sarah Gebauer, Ph.D., is a nutritionist in the Office of Nutrition and Food Labeling, Center for Food Safety and Applied Nutrition, at the U.S. Food and Drug Administration (FDA). She works in the Nutrition Science Review Branch where she reviews the scientific evidence related to nutrition labeling and label claims (e.g., health claims, nutrient content claims). Dr. Gebauer helped implement the FDA regulatory definition of dietary fiber and reviews

the evidence to determine whether isolated or synthetic nondigestible carbohydrates meet the regulatory definition of dietary fiber. She is a member
of the U.S.-Canada Joint Dietary Reference Intakes (DRIs) Working Group
involved with the process to update the DRIs for energy, protein, carbohy-
drate, and fat. Prior to joining FDA, Dr. Gebauer worked at the Beltsville
Human Nutrition Research Center, Agricultural Research Service, at the
U.S. Department of Agriculture, where she conducted highly controlled
dietary interventions to investigate the relationship between food/food
components and risk of chronic diseases, such as cardiovascular disease and
diabetes. She received a B.S. in biology and a Ph.D. in molecular medicine,
both from Penn State University.

Lee Hooper, Ph.D., R.D., is a reader in research synthesis, nutrition, and
hydration in the Norwich Medical School at the University of East Anglia
and has a B.Sc. in biochemistry, Ph.D. (University of Manchester), and is a
registered dietitian. She worked as a dietitian in the National Health Service
for 10 years, with extensive experience of community health promotion and
cardiovascular health. Dr. Hooper moved to research in 2000 and has since
published more than 100 peer-reviewed publications, mainly in the areas of
dehydration and nutrition of older people and the effects of dietary change
on health. Her publications have been cited more than 30,000 times with
an h-index of 82. Dr. Hooper has a long-term interest in the nutrition and
hydration of older people. She is an expert systematic reviewer and has
developed and managed numerous systematic reviews. Dr. Hooper was an
editor for the Cochrane Heart Group for 14 years, was an editor of the
Cochrane Oral Health Group for 5 years, and regularly referees systematic
reviews for top medical and nutrition journals.

Andrew Jones, Ph.D., is a senior lecturer in psychology at Liverpool John
Moores University. He is an experimental psychologist with a wider interest
in meta-science and evidence syntheses. His research focuses on the ante-
cedents and consequences of unhealthy behaviors, such as alcohol use and
poor dietary choices. He has received early career awards from the British
Association for Psychopharmacology and Society for the Study of Addic-
tion. He has authored more than 100 journal articles and received funding
from the National Institute for Health and Care Research, the Economic
and Social Research Council, and Public Health England.

Amanda J. MacFarlane, Ph.D., is the founding director of the Agriculture,
Food, and Nutrition Evidence Center and Professor of Nutrition at Texas
A&M University (2022–present). Her research examines the impact of
B-vitamin nutrition on health spanning the molecular mechanisms under-
pinning genome stability to the identification of socioeconomic, dietary,

and genetic determinants of population nutritional status. She is a member of the NuQuest Working Group that developed critical appraisal tools for nutrition studies. While a research scientist at Health Canada (2008–2022), she chaired the Canada—U.S. Joint Dietary Reference Intakes (DRIs) Working Group (2013–2022), during which time chronic disease endpoints were formally included in the DRIs framework, the sodium and potassium DRIs were reviewed, and a review of macronutrient requirements was initiated. She is actively involved in policy work related to food fortification, food labeling, and vitamin supplements. She is an associate editor of *The American Journal of Clinical Nutrition* and member-at-large for food and nutrition policy of the Board of Directors of the American Society for Nutrition. She received the 2022 Assistant Deputy Minister's Award for Excellence in Science, the 2017 Deputy Minister's Award for Excellence in Science, and the 2015 Assistant Deputy Minister's Award for Transparency and Openness. Dr. MacFarlane received her B.Sc. in biology and biotechnology from Carleton University in 2000 and her Ph.D. in biochemistry from the University of Ottawa in 2004. Dr. MacFarlane is a member of the Scientific Advisory Group for the Bill & Melinda Gates Foundation–funded Micronutrient International project "Development and Market Introduction of Iodine-Folic Acid Fortified Salt (DFS-IoFA) in Ethiopia" from 2023 to present. Dr. MacFarlane serves in uncompensated roles as a guest member of the World Health Organization Obesity Technical Working Group from 2022 to present; the Director-at-Large of Food and Nutrition Policy, American Society for Nutrition Board of Directors from 2021 to present; a member of the European Food Safety Authority Expert Panel for hazard identification of folate/folic acid in 2021; the chair of the Joint Canada-U.S. Dietary Reference Intakes Working Group from 2013–2022; a member of the Scientific Advisory Group for the Nordic Nutrition Recommendations 2022 from 2019 to present; and member of the Canadian Nutrition Society Ethics Committee from 2018 to present. She has served as an associate editor for *The American Journal of Clinical Nutrition* since 2018.

Vasanti Malik, Sc.D., is an assistant professor in the Department of Nutritional Sciences, Temerty Faculty of Medicine at the University of Toronto, and an adjunct assistant professor in the Department of Nutrition at the Harvard T.H. Chan School of Public Health. She holds a Canada Research Chair in Nutrition and Chronic Disease Prevention. Dr. Malik's research uses a combination of epidemiological studies, clinical trials, and evidence synthesis to evaluate dietary and lifestyle determinants of obesity and cardiometabolic diseases in different populations and across the life course. Dr. Malik's research also includes studying the intersection of diet, health, and environmental sustainability with the goal of informing dietary guidance and public policies to prevent chronic diseases and promote more sustainable food systems.

M. Hassan Murad, Ph.D., is an epidemiologist and professor of medicine at the Mayo Clinic with a career focus on improving the methods of evidence synthesis, translation and integration in practice, policy, and guidelines. He directs the Agency for Healthcare Research and Quality–designated Evidence-based Practice Center at the Mayo Clinic, the fellowship program in preventive medicine and public health, and the master's program in translational research. He is a cofounder of the US-GRADE Network, has more than 950 scientific publications, and participated in more than 80 national/international practice guidelines.

Celeste Naude, Ph.D., M.Nutr., R.D., is an associate professor and chief researcher at the Centre for Evidence-based Health Care, Department of Global Health, Stellenbosch University, South Africa (SA); and codirector of Cochrane Nutrition. Her academic interests and experience include health and nutrition evidence synthesis and evidence-informed decision making in policy and practice for improving nutrition, health, and other sustainable development outcomes. Dr. Naude is involved in producing systematic reviews and other evidence syntheses for the World Health Organization's (WHO's) guideline development processes. She also serves as a member of the WHO Nutrition Guidance Expert Advisory Group Subgroup on Policy Actions, and as a guideline methodologist for WHO nutrition guidelines. She is involved in international, regional, and national research and policy partnerships and networks. She leads the nutrition focus area of the Research, Evidence and Development Initiative, funded by UK aid from the UK government, and the evidence synthesis work package for the Global Evidence, Local Adaptation project in South Africa, funded by European and Developing Countries Clinical Trials Partnership, which focuses on newborn and child health guidelines in South Africa, Malawi, and Nigeria. Dr. Naude has served on the South Africa Ministerial Committee on Mortality and Morbidity in Children, as an associate editor of the Cochrane Effective Practice and Organization of Care Group, as cochair of the Cochrane Council and Fields Executive, and as a member of the WHO/Cochrane Working Group. She is a member of the South Africa Grading of Recommendations Assessment, Development and Evaluation Network and on the Advisory Group for the Enabling sustainable public engagement in improving health and health equity (IHC CHOICE) project, led by the Norwegian Institute of Public Health.

Sydne J. Newberry, Ph.D., has served as a project lead, literature reviewer, and medical editor for the Southern California Evidence-based Practice Center, formerly based at the RAND Corporation, since 2000. She has conducted and participated in evidence reviews in the areas of nutrition and metabolism, endocrinology, military health, integrative medicine, and other areas of clinical medicine. Topics of recent reviews have included the health effects of dietary sodium and potassium, the effects of omega-3 fatty acids in maternal and child health, the effects of omega-3 fatty acids in treating major depressive disorder, the health effects of vitamin D, and the comparative effectiveness of treatments for low bone density and osteoporosis—all conducted for the Agency for Healthcare Research and Quality or the Department of Defense. Prior to joining RAND, she was a nutrition instructor and project manager for the Department of Community Health Sciences in the University of California, Los Angeles (UCLA), School of Public Health, managing the editing and revision of a nutrition encyclopedia for consumers and a reproductive nutrition guide for healthcare providers. Prior to joining UCLA, she was a project officer for the Institute of Medicine/Food and Nutrition Board/Committee on Military Nutrition Research of the National Academy of Sciences. Dr. Newberry has also held academic and research positions at the Ohio State University (OSU) and the Fels Research Institute/Wright State University School of Medicine (Dayton, Ohio) and has worked as a clinical nutritionist in hospital-based weight management clinics. She received her Ph.D. in nutritional biochemistry and metabolism (minor in neuroendocrinology) at the Massachusetts Institute of Technology and completed postdoctoral work in molecular and cellular biology and plant virology at OSU.

Chizuru Nishida, Ph.D., after serving as the coordinator (head) of Nutrition Policy and Scientific Advice Unit of the World Health Organization (WHO) Department of Nutrition for Health and Development for 10 years, served as the Head of the Cross-Cutting Unit of Safe, Healthy and Sustainable Diet at the newly merged WHO Department of Nutrition and Food Safety from 2020 to 2023. She continued to lead the development of WHO guidance and scientific advice on diet, nutrition, and health before she retired at the end of February 2023 from WHO, where she worked for almost 36 years at all three levels (global, regional, and county level) of the Organization. Dr. Nishida also served as the head of a WHO delegation at the Codex Committees on Nutrition and Food for Special Dietary Uses and Food Labelling for the last 20 years, leading and ensuring policy coherence in the development of Codex standards and guidelines not only to protect food safety but also to improve food quality to address increasing global public health problems of obesity and diet-related noncommunicable diseases. During 2019–2023, she served as the chair of the Cochrane Nutrition Advisory Board, which guided the work and strategic direction of Cochrane Nutrition. She received the Asia Pacific Clinical Nutrition Society Award for 2023. Dr. Nishida holds a Ph.D. in nutrition science and an M.A. in medical anthropology.

Crystal Rivers, M.S., is a nutritionist in the Office of Nutrition and Food Labeling, Center for Food Safety and Applied Nutrition, U.S. Food and Drug Administration (FDA). She is a member of the Nutrition Science Review Branch that is responsible for the premarket review of scientific evidence for health claims. She also works on issues related to the Nutrition Facts label. Prior to joining FDA in 2005, Rivers worked as a research associate at the Institute of Medicine's Food and Nutrition Board on the Dietary Reference Intakes (DRIs). She was also an extension agent with Virginia Cooperative Extension, where she taught educational programs in nutrition and food safety. Rivers holds a B.S. and an M.S. in human nutrition, foods and exercise from Virginia Polytechnic Institute and State University (Virginia Tech).

Christopher Schmid, Ph.D., is professor of biostatistics and founding member of the Center for Evidence Synthesis in Health in the Brown School of Public Health at Brown University. Dr. Schmid also directs the Biostatistics, Epidemiology, and Research Design Core of Advance-RI Clinical and Translational Research and the Evidence Synthesis Academy. His research focuses on methods and applications for meta-analysis, particularly Bayesian methods and software on predictive models derived from combining data from different sources and on clinical trials, particularly N-of-1 trials, and single person multiple crossover studies. Dr. Schmid received his Ph.D. in statistics from Harvard University.

Barbara O. Schneeman, Ph.D., is emeritus professor of nutrition at the University of California, Davis. From 2004 to 2013 she was the director of the Office of Nutrition, Labeling, and Dietary Supplements at the U.S. Food and Drug Administration. She chaired the 2020 Dietary Guidelines Advisory Committee and served on the 1990 and 1995 Committees. She is a member of two nutrition advisory committees for the World Health Organization and a member of the National Academies of Sciences, Engineering, and Medicine's Food and Nutrition Board. Dr. Schneeman has received several awards and has been recognized for her work on dietary fiber, gastrointestinal function, development and use of food-based dietary guidelines, and policy development in food and nutrition. She is a fellow of the American Society for Nutrition and the American Association for the Advancement of Science.

Janet A. Tooze, Ph.D., M.P.H., is a professor in the Department of Biostatistics and Data Science, Division of Public Health Sciences, Wake Forest University School of Medicine. She is a biostatistician with expertise in statistical methods in nutrition, focused on dietary assessment and measurement error. She has developed methods for estimating the usual intake of foods and nutrients in a unified framework, termed the NCI Method, the foundation of which is a statistical model developed by Dr. Tooze for repeated measures data with excess zeroes. This method is used internationally to characterize population intakes of foods and nutrients and for risk assessment. Dr. Tooze received an M.P.H. from the Harvard School of Public Health and a Ph.D. from the University of Colorado. She was a member of the 2017–2019 Committee to Review the Dietary Intakes for Sodium and Potassium and the 2021–2022 Committee to Review the Dietary Intakes for Energy for the National Academies of Sciences, Engineering, and Medicine. She led the statistical validation of the Healthy Eating Index-2015, a widely used diet quality index, and the Total Nutrient Index. She has received three National Institutes of Health Merit Awards in recognition of her work in the advancement of dietary assessment.

Katherine L. Tucker, Ph.D., is University Distinguished Professor of Nutritional Epidemiology in the Department of Biomedical and Nutrition Sciences and director of the Center for Population Health, at the University of Massachusetts Lowell. She holds an adjunct appointment at the University of Massachusetts Medical School. Before joining UMass Lowell, she was at the U.S. Department of Agriculture Human Nutrition Research Center on Aging at Tufts University and McGill University. Dr. Tucker has contributed to more than 450 articles in scientific journals. Her research focuses on dietary intake and risk of chronic disease, including osteoporosis, cognitive decline, obesity, metabolic syndrome, and heart disease with an emphasis on health disparities. She is the principal investigator of the Boston Puerto Rican Health Study, an ongoing cohort study, to examine the roles of diet, health behaviors, stress, and genetic predisposition in relation to chronic conditions, including heart disease, cognitive decline, and bone health. She is actively involved as a scientific advisor for the National Heart, Lung, and Blood Institute's Jackson Heart Study and served two terms on the Food and Nutrition Board of the National Academies of Sciences, Engineering, and Medicine. She is a fellow of the American Society for Nutrition (ASN), the Gerontological Society of America, and the American Society for Bone Mineral Research. She is currently the editor-in-chief of *Advances in Nutrition*, the international review journal of the ASN and senior editor of the forthcoming 12th edition of the textbook *Modern Nutrition in Health and Disease*. She received her Ph.D. from Cornell University and her undergraduate degree from the University of Connecticut, both in nutritional sciences.

George A. Wells, Ph.D., M.Sc., is a professor in the School of Epidemiology and Public Health at the University of Ottawa and director of the Cardiovascular Research Methods Centre at the University of Ottawa Heart Institute. He is also a professor in the Department of Medicine at the

University of Ottawa. His research interests are in the design and analysis of clinical trials, health technology assessment, statistical methodology related to health care delivery, systematic reviews and meta-analysis, economic evaluations, and the development and assessment of decision support technologies for patients and practitioners. Dr. Wells is the author or coauthor of more than 900 peer-reviewed articles and more than 1,000 scientific abstracts. He has been the principal investigator or co-investigator on more than 310 research projects.